FIT FOR GOOD

DISCOVERING THE CONNECTION BETWEEN PHYSICAL AND SPIRITUAL STRENGTH

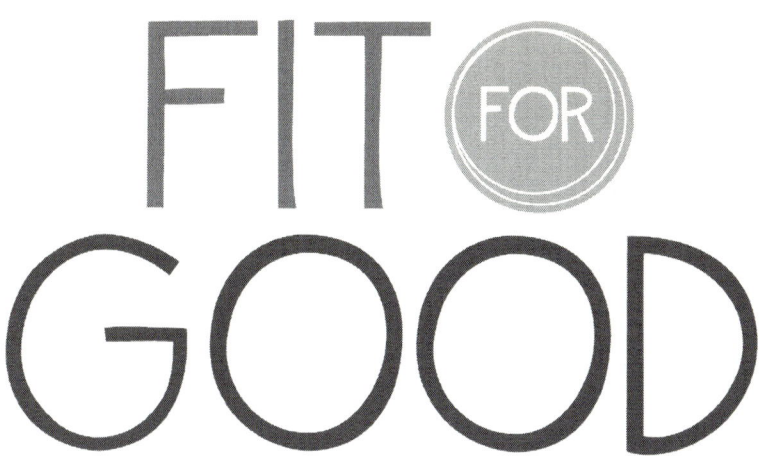

DISCOVERING THE CONNECTION BETWEEN
PHYSICAL AND SPIRITUAL STRENGTH

DR. H. RICH TENNEY
AND LIZ TENNYSON

CFI, an imprint of Cedar Fort, Inc.
Springville, Utah

© 2017 Dr. H. Rich Tenney and Liz Tennyson
All rights reserved.

No part of this book may be reproduced in any form whatsoever, whether by graphic, visual, electronic, film, microfilm, tape recording, or any other means, without prior written permission of the publisher, except in the case of brief passages embodied in critical reviews and articles.

This is not an official publication of The Church of Jesus Christ of Latter-day Saints. The opinions and views expressed herein belong solely to the author and do not necessarily represent the opinions or views of Cedar Fort, Inc. Permission for the use of sources, graphics, and photos is also solely the responsibility of the author.

The material in this book is for informational purposes only. Please ensure you are safe to exercise and safe when you exercise by consulting with your health care practitioner before beginning any exercise program.

ISBN 13: 978-1-4621-1974-5

Published by CFI an imprint of Cedar Fort, Inc., 2373 W. 700 S., Springville, UT 84663
Distributed by Cedar Fort, Inc., www.cedarfort.com

LIBRARY OF CONGRESS CATALOGING-IN-PUBLICATION DATA

Names: Tenney, H. Rich, 1976- author. | Tennyson, Liz, 1978- author.
Title: Fit for good / Dr. H. Rich Tenney and Liz Tennyson.
Description: Springville, Utah : CFI, An imprint of Cedar Fort, Inc., [2016] | Includes bibliographical references and index.
Identifiers: LCCN 2016052411 (print) | LCCN 2016053232 (ebook) | ISBN 9781462119745 (perfect bound : alk. paper) | ISBN 9781462127450 (epub, pdf, mobi)
Subjects: LCSH: Health--Religious aspects--Church of Jesus Christ of Latter-day Saints. | Health--Religious aspects--Mormon Church. | Physical fitness--Religious aspects--Church of Jesus Christ of Latter-day Saints. | Physical fitness--Religious aspects--Mormon Church.
Classification: LCC BX8643.H8 T46 2016 (print) | LCC BX8643.H8 (ebook) | DDC 248.4/89332--dc23
LC record available at https://lccn.loc.gov/2016052411

Cover design by Shawnda T. Craig
Cover design © 2017 by Cedar Fort, Inc.
Edited and typeset by Chelsea Holdaway

Printed in the United States of America

10 9 8 7 6 5 4 3 2 1

Printed on acid-free paper

Dedicated to Tami—my perfect fit.
Dr. H. Rich Tenney

To my husband and children who are patient and kind and accept me with my crazy radical ideas. I love you all so much.
Liz Tennyson

CONTENTS

Preface ix
Introduction xv

PART ONE: ON YOUR MARKS — 1

Chapter 1: Receive the Measure of Your Creation 3
Chapter 2: Yoke Yourself to the Power of Godliness 13
Chapter 3: Consecrate to Be Quickened 25

PART TWO: GET SET — 33

Chapter 4: By the Sweat of Your Brow 35
Chapter 5: Defend against the Adversary's Fiery Darts 47
Chapter 6: Experiment upon the Word of God 59

PART THREE: GO! — 69

Chapter 7: Create a Fitness Focus 71
Chapter 8: Form Your Flesh 89
Chapter 9: Divide the Light from the Darkness Within 107
Chapter 10: Beautify Your Fitness 125
Chapter 11: Multiply the Blessings 143
Chapter 12: Become Fit for Good 157

Notes 171
Personal Notes 177
About the Author: Dr. H. Rich Tenney 187
About the Author: Liz Tennyson 189

PREFACE

As you read this book, you will hear from two perspectives. Much of this book is from the original *Fit for Good* text written by Dr. H. Rich Tenney. His insights, studies, and perspectives are amazing. He'll teach you powerful gospel principles and common ways to apply them in everyday life. Throughout the book you will also read stories from me, Liz Tennyson. I have a quirky and energetic personality, but I'm solid in my spiritual gifts and my deep love for my brothers and sisters in Christ. This preface is meant to help you realize the importance of the book, how it came to pass, and the reason *you* are reading it now.

In 2010, I went through a massive transformation in my own life—a transformation that humbled and guided me to a new testimony and a new life of wanting to be a better disciple.

At this time, I was listening to "Help Them on Their Way Home" by President Henry B. Eyring.

"Heavenly Father has assigned us to a great variety of stations to strengthen and, when needed, to lead travelers to safety."[1] I started weeping as I felt the Spirit pierce my heart with a new assignment from my Heavenly Father. I had become a runner while on a previous weight-loss journey. I felt like I actually ran out of darkness and despair and into light and hope. As I heard him talk about "stations," I thought about the many

Preface

water stations available while running a marathon. Sometimes I would stop to drink because I was really thirsty. Sometimes I would just grab and go because I just needed a quick sip. Whatever the case, I appreciated the support of those water stations, and I wanted to provide that support to others. This has become my life mission: to help others as they run their sometimes physical—but more often metaphorical—marathon of life.

When I was a young girl, I had a great leader who taught me that my calling would come in many ways—and not just when I was specifically called to a formal calling at church. There would be times when I would be assigned to one person on the street, or to many people as I spoke, or to my children in my roles as a mother and wife. (I got to choose these assignments.) I remembered that wisdom as I began my new calling as a life coach. In this new calling, I would get an opportunity to testify that God lives, that He is our Father, and that we have an advocate through the Savior to fulfill our assignments both here and in heaven. This has all been manifested to me in lessons of the physical body and this earthly experience. President Dieter F. Uchtdorf said,

> The truth is, those who diligently seek to learn of Christ eventually will come to know Him. They will personally receive a divine portrait of the Master, although it most often comes in the form of a puzzle—one piece at a time. Each individual piece may not be easily recognizable by itself; it may not be clear how it relates to the whole. Each piece helps us to see the big picture a little more clearly. Eventually, after enough pieces have been put together, we recognize the grand beauty of it all. Then, looking back on our experience, we see that the Savior had indeed come to be with us—not all at once but quietly, gently, almost unnoticed.[2]

That experience I had while listening to President Eyring's talk inspired me to change my course in life. Since that time, I have been a personal trainer and certified holistic health and life coach for many years. I have studied and received much training on different ways to teach and share the message I have with others. I have helped thousands of women and families gain a new perspective. I am just a friend that has been given the opportunity to hand you my cup of water as you run this marathon of

Preface

life—whether you're thirsty or just need to dump it over your head to get to the next station in your race. I pray that you will give me permission to share candidly and openly the amazing experiences that our Heavenly Father has blessed me with and to open your eyes and ears to the evidence that He wants the same for you. You are loved. In the last ten years, I have gained this testimony. I hope to serve my small assignment with grace. I pray that your mind may be clear and your heart open to the Spirit as you realize that you also have been assigned to achieve amazing things and that your physical body *will* help you. I also understand the limitations you may have. I invite you to realize that you can use *all* things for good. You can choose joy, build a solid testimony on the lessons that you get to experience, and experiment with your individual limitation.

I'm excited to share my experiences with you side by side with Dr. H. Rich Tenney, who has had his own journey of becoming *fit for good.*

A simple spring-loaded tape measure—that's what started the *Fit for Good* journey for me.

I remember as a young boy wandering into the garage to rummage through my father's toolbox. That spring-loaded tape measure caught my attention. I had seen my father unleash its impressive recoil many a time in the garden and on his workbench. I quickly grabbed it and ran to the living room. After pulling and releasing it several times, a simple question entered my mind. *I wonder how tall I am?* I locked the tape measure and laid down next to it. I eyeballed my heels and then placed a finger on the tape measure in line with the top of my head. After standing up, I looked at the length of my body and thought to myself, *I'm short!*

That experience ignited my passion for the human body and led me on my path to become a doctor of physical therapy. Over the last ten years, I've had the opportunity to work with thousands of patients in an effort to help them understand and move their bodies in ways that can relieve their pain and improve their performance.

However, there's an underlying problem with my profession. I'm financially forced to treat my patients reactively—meaning after disease

Preface

and dysfunction have already set in. This approach keeps me busy, but it does little to address the primary problem—life *behaviors* that cause my patients' bodies to breakdown.

In physical therapy, behavior change is the goal. Therapists are always looking for and developing new tools and techniques that will positively influence our patients' movement and lifestyle behaviors. In the beginning of my practice, I quickly discovered that though these tools or techniques are important, my patients' motivation has the greatest impact on whether treatment is successful or not.

Knowing this, I began to look for motivational principles, patterns, and practices that I could implement to help my patients experience lasting change in their fitness behavior. I read the best books, studied the most recent research, and contemplated the guidelines given by the most notable motivational gurus.

Then I read this well-known quote given by President Boyd K. Packer with new eyes: "The study of the doctrines of the gospel will improve behavior quicker than a study of behavior will improve behavior. . . . That is why we stress so forcefully the study of the doctrines of the gospel."[3]

I knew that there was nothing more powerful than the doctrine found in the gospel to help an individual improve their health behaviors. I dove into the scriptures and the words of the prophets, looking for specific principles, patterns, and practices that could help an individual improve their health behaviors for good. After three years of study and writing I finished the first edition of *Fit for Good*. Six months later, a Facebook friend shared with me a post by #Imafitmormon. The name of the post alone set my heart racing. After reading the post, I knew I had to reach out to whoever was behind this.

That's when I got an nonrandom email from Dr. Tenney. He had written this amazing book called *Fit for Good* and wanted to know if I would read it. At the time, I was not open to reading the book, but I *was* open to having a phone call to understand more about his intention for reaching out. We had a great conversation about his book, and I decided to read it when I had time.

Preface

Little did I know that he had also been assigned with some very familiar teachings and information. As I read his book, it was another confirmation that Heavenly Father clearly wanted this message to be shared. As I continued to read, I learned of principles and practices I hadn't thought of before. My eyes were opening and my heart was full.

We have been very excited to have partnered together as we combine our ideas in this new version of *Fit for Good*.

President Uchtdorf said, "It has been my experience that some of the most powerful promptings we receive are not only for our own benefit but also for the benefit of others. If we are thinking only of ourselves, we may miss some of the most powerful spiritual experiences and profound revelations of our lives."[4]

Our intention is to help our brothers and sisters gain more knowledge as we try to help the Spirit deliver our perspective on the heavenly messages we want to share. We hope to help you on your path of discipleship and your physical marathon here on earth.

INTRODUCTION

My chest felt like it was going to explode. I struggled to pull in the hot, dry Arizona air as the intense pumping of my heart sent uncomfortable shock waves throughout my body. I could see a large amount of concern, sprinkled with a little frustration, on my wife's face. "Honey, you didn't have to run," she whispered as she gently wiped my forehead.

My wife was right; I didn't have to run the Fourth of July Boot Race, but I was thirty years old! My younger age undoubtedly gave me the advantage in the thirty to thirty-five age bracket. It would be another six years before I'd have that advantage again. I was confident I could win the race. I had won it before when I was a strong eighteen-year-old just out of high school. So against my wife's good counsel, and with the confidence and mentality of an eighteen-year-old, I decided to take my thirty-year-old, out-of-shape body and a pair of old cowboy boots for a sprint down the one hundred yards of asphalt the locals called "Whiskey Row."

"Runners to your mark!" yelled the starter as he raised his gun into the air. I stepped to the starting mark and dug my cowboy boots into the pavement as best I could. My plaid shorts flapped in the wind as I peered through my sunglasses at the one hundred yards of hot, unforgiving asphalt ahead. Thousands of spectators looked on as the starter yelled, "Get set!" My body tensed as I crouched in anticipation. . . . BANG! The

Introduction

starter fired the gun. I burst off the line. It was a great start! Within a few quick strides, I found myself at the front of the pack. I was giddy; I had a shot at winning the race! In my mind, I could hear my high school track coach telling me to stay relaxed and keep my form as I accelerated toward the finish line. The sound of the other runners' cowboy boots began to fade behind me as I ran like I was eighteen . . . for exactly seventy of the one hundred yards. That's when reality slammed me into my thirty-year-old, out-of-shape body.

Instantly my legs transformed into a pair of partially cooked noodles. My arms began to flail, trying to keep my legs from buckling. My eyes burned, and my vision blurred from the salty sweat pouring down from my bald head. In my moment of body breakdown, the finish line now looked like a mirage more than a mile away. My priorities quickly changed. My desire to win was quickly replaced by my desire to finish without a crash that would send me forever into the oral history of my future family reunions. I slowed my pace significantly and stumbled toward the finish line, but within only five yards of the finish line, two of my competitors passed me.

I crossed the line and bent over, braying like a donkey, trying to catch my breath. The race coordinators ushered the finishers to the side. I propped myself up on the shoulder of the winner, wheezed out a congratulations, and then headed straight for the lawn next to the courthouse, trying to keep my lunch from coming up. For the next thirty minutes, I lay still and tried to recover from my physical breakdown while my wife threatened to call the paramedics. On the way home, I made a commitment to myself that I was going to get fit for the next race—when I turned thirty-six, of course.

Each of us has had experiences that reveal the measure of our physical fitness. The most common reminders come in the form of a flight of stairs that seem to send us into cardiac arrest, or a young child that points at a picture of you from just a few years back and asks, "Who's that next to Mommy?" However, the more powerful measures come from the honest mirror, the weight scale, or the medical professional that paints a serious

Introduction

picture with our lab results. These common reminders stir millions of people to spend billions of dollars each year in hopes of improving their physical fitness. There are those whose fitness efforts become a reality, and they experience great success as witnessed by their amazing physical transformations on TV, on the Internet, and in magazines. However, they are the minority when compared to the millions who have tried again and again to get and stay fit to no avail.

Why do we fail so often at our efforts to get fit and stay fit? Scientists, health professionals, and public officials have spent vast amounts of money and have devoted much time trying to figure out how to motivate us to improve our fitness behaviors. However, each year, the research reveals little to no change in our fitness success.[1] Is there "a more excellent way" (1 Corinthians 12:31) to improve our physical fitness? There is. President Boyd K. Packer tells us that the way comes from understanding true doctrine, for "true doctrine, understood" can improve our behavior—including our fitness behavior—"quicker than a study of behavior will."[2]

This book aims to help you improve your fitness behaviors for good by helping you understand and then act upon true doctrines of the gospel as they relate to your physical body. Doctrine, when understood, will help you overcome fitness failure and enable you to become physically *fit for good*.

Part one, titled "On Your Marks," will help you "mark" the doctrine that will measure, yoke, and quicken your efforts to get physically fit. Part two, titled "Get Set," will help you prepare for the physical sweat and the fiery darts of the adversary who will fight your efforts to get fit. This section will also prepare you to experiment upon the word of God to assist your efforts in becoming physically fit. Part three, titled "Go!," will help you understand and act upon our Father in Heaven's pattern of physical creation—to form, divide, beautify, and multiply your physical fitness efforts: the eternal pattern that will enable you to *become* physically *fit for good*.

I want to prepare you up front. This book is *not* intended to be one you can casually read and then put back on your real or electronic bookshelf. It is not an exercise routine that promises a better-looking body

Introduction

by exercising twenty minutes per day, three days a week. However, it is a book that can help you understand and then act upon gospel doctrine that will inspire you to get, and stay, physically *fit for good* (meaning fit to do good, forever, like our Savior). This book will invite you to learn "precept upon precept; line upon line" (Isaiah 28:10) how to "exercise" dominion over the elements of your body and enable you to fill the measure of your creation with a fulness of joy.

PART ONE
On Your Marks

At the beginning of my failed boot race, the starter prepared the runners with this command: "Runners, to your mark!" All races are composed of three marks: the mark that starts the race, the mark that outlines the path, and the mark that finishes the race. Now consider how critical these marks are to runners. The starting mark, or the starting line, provides runners with a reference point that reveals the measured distance required to finish the race. The mark that outlines the path to the finishing line gives runners purpose and direction. The final mark, or the finish line, signals to runners that they have met their goal. Without these marks, the race would fail to exist because it would have no beginning and therefore no end. What you choose as your fitness marks will ultimately determine your fitness success. The next three chapters will help you understand and step up to the eternal marks that will *measure*, *yoke*, and *quicken* your efforts to get and stay physically *fit for good*.

CHAPTER 1

Receive the Measure of Your Creation

A few years ago, I attended a college football game with my father and my two older brothers. I don't recall much of the game, but there is one experience from that day I will always remember. We were leaving the stadium, and for some reason I became distracted and fell behind my family members. I quickened my pace to catch up; however, rather than immediately joining my father and brothers, I tarried behind and watched them walk and converse together. I found joy in watching them interact as they used various hand gestures and body postures to express themselves. Within a few moments, I began to focus on their gait, or walking patterns—a habit formed from a career in physical therapy.

I saw something amazing that brought a smile to my face. In front of me were three grown men walking in near perfect unison. Their right feet slightly turned out with each step as their left arms swung forward, combined with a little shoulder drop on the right to bring it all together. If there was such a thing as synchronized walking in the Olympics, my father and brothers would have been gold medal favorites. Maybe you have had an experience like this while watching a home video of your parents and noticing how much you look, sound, and even act like them. Maybe you said to yourself, "I'm turning into my mother!" or "I sound so much like my father!"

I continued to hover behind my father and brothers, amazed by the consistent unison of their movement. As I watched them, I began to experience an overwhelming feeling of great love for my father and brothers in their physical unity. The Spirit whispered to my mind, "Look! Your brothers have been made in the image of your Father!" At that moment, I felt a profound sense of closeness to my father and my brothers. I quickly ran to join them.

A few years later as I was exiting the same stadium with thousands of fans following another football game, the Spirit whispered again, "Look! They too have been made in the image of their Father; they are His children." That experience reminded me of a scripture: "And God said, Let us make man in our image, after our likeness. . . . So God created man in his *own* image, in the image of God created he him; male and female created he them" (Genesis 1:26–27; italics in original). I felt as if I were on sacred ground as I watched and walked with thousands of God's children, my brothers and sisters, exiting the stadium in the image of their Father.

MEASURED

Let's transition from a stadium to an exceedingly high mountain with the prophet Moses to deepen our understanding of what it means to be made in the image of God. On this mountain, Moses was blessed to see not just some of Heavenly Father's children, but all of them that were and ever will be upon the earth. "And it came to pass that Moses looked, and beheld the world upon which he was created; and Moses beheld the world and the ends thereof, and all the children of men which are, and which were created; *of the same* he greatly marveled and wondered" (Moses 1:8; emphasis added). Focus your thoughts on the phrase "of the same" within this verse. What was *the same* about all the children of men that caused Moses to marvel and wonder? Some previous verses provide the answer.

Prior to showing Moses all of His children, our Father in Heaven revealed to Moses the "I am" doctrine of who He really is. "Behold, *I am* the Lord God Almighty, and Endless is my name; for *I am* without

Receive the Measure of Your Creation

beginning of days or end of years; and is not this *endless*?" (Moses 1:3; emphasis added). The "I am" doctrine of God points toward His endless nature, and His endless nature is the eternal measure of God's existence—the way He views Himself. With this established in Moses's mind, our Father in Heaven then revealed to Moses the *measure* of Moses's, and our, creation. The Father first declared the well-known "thou art" doctrine of Moses's spiritual identity, saying, "behold, *thou art* my son" (Moses 1:4; emphasis added). The Father then revealed the *measure* of Moses's physical creation, the "thou art" doctrine of his physical identity, saying, "Moses, my son . . . *thou art* in the similitude of mine Only Begotten" (Moses 1:6; emphasis added).

What did this mean, to be in the similitude of God's Only Begotten Son? We can gain a better understanding of this doctrine in the confrontation that Moses had with Satan following this revelation. After the presence of God withdrew from Moses, Satan came, tempting him with this command: "Moses, *son of man*, worship me" (Moses 1:12; emphasis added).

Now consider what thoughts might have been going through Moses's mind after hearing this command. He had just communed face-to-face with his Father, the almighty God, who had declared to him the "thou art" doctrine of his spiritual and physical identity. Moses knew that he was a *spiritual* son of God who was created *physically* in the similitude of God's Only Begotten Son. Knowing this, "Moses looked upon Satan" (Moses 1:13) and *measured* him against what he had just seen and learned from his Father in Heaven. He boldly questioned Satan:

"Who art thou? For behold, . . ."	*(In other words, look at me.)*
"I am a son of God, in the similitude of His Only Begotten . . ."	*(I am a spiritual son of God that has a body of flesh and bones similar to the Father's Only Begotten Son.)*
"Where is thy glory that I should worship thee?" (Moses 1:13).	*(You are without physical form.)*

Fit for Good

"Wherefore I can judge between him . . ."	*(God is a glorious, exalted, physical being.)*
"And thee."	*(You are a spirit only.)*
"Depart hence, Satan" (Moses 1:18).	

Satan was infuriated by Moses's bold measurement of his disembodied state. "Rant[ing] upon the earth," he commanded Moses to worship him, declaring that he was the only begotten. Seeing Satan's power, Moses began to fear. He called upon the name of God, whom he was physically made in similitude of, and commanded Satan to depart (Moses 1:19–22).

The Apostle Paul declared this doctrine of our physical identity on Mars Hill in Athens, Greece. When teaching the citizens of Athens the correct idea of God's physical attributes, he declared, "*He be not far* from every one of us: For in him we *live*, and *move*, and *have our being*; as certain also of your own poets have said, For we *are also his offspring*. Forasmuch then as we are the offspring of God, we ought not think that the Godhead is like unto gold, or silver, or stone, graven by art and man's device" (Acts 17:27–29; emphasis added).

Paul taught that God is not physically far from us. We are His offspring. We live, move, and have our being, a physical body, like Him! Brigham Young stated, "When we look upon the human face *we look upon the image of our Father* and God; there is a divinity in each person, male and female, there is the heavenly, there is the divine."[1]

What a powerful doctrine! Whenever you look at another individual's physical being, you are looking at the image of God's physical being. How different would our world be if we all could consistently see God in others and ourselves? Knowing that you are physically made in God's image is the first eternal doctrine that, when marked and "stepped toward," will motivate you to get and stay physically *fit for good*. We can step to this mark by answering the question posed by the prophet Alma when he asked the people of Zarahemla, "have ye *received* his image in your countenances?" (Alma 5:14; emphasis added).

Receive the Measure of Your Creation

Alma indicates that we can act to *receive* God's image, and that when we do, His image will be manifested in our countenances. Sister Elaine S. Dalton, while serving in the Relief Society general presidency, shared an experience of a young woman receiving the image of God during a visit to her office:

> Recently, a group of young women visited my office. At the end of the visit, one young woman confided with tears in her eyes, "I have never thought of myself as beautiful. I have always felt very ordinary. But today, as I walked past the mirror in your office and glanced into it, I was beautiful!" She *was* beautiful because her face shone with the Spirit. *She saw herself as our Heavenly Father sees her* [emphasis added]. She had *received* His image in her countenance [emphasis added].[2]

We can receive God's image when we "learn to see [ourselves] as Heavenly Father sees [us]—as His precious daughter[s] or son[s] with divine potential."[3] Learning to see ourselves as God sees us is more than just knowing that we are His spirit children. It includes knowing that our physical bodies *are the measure* of our physical creation—the physical evidence of our divine potential to become like God.

As a young mother, I visited a friend who had just had a baby. As I was holding the small baby, who was only a couple of hours old, the Spirit taught me a truth that would be become a deep part of my belief system and how I conducted myself. I learned that the body is an important part of our Heavenly Father's plan. In heaven, we shouted for joy as we heard about this body we would receive. Our Heavenly Father is consistent, and I believe He was candid about our experience here. He explained to us what an amazing creation our bodies would be and how they would be created for our success. We said, "Yes! I want a body. Yes! I want to go."

When we come here, we come as a baby. In our simplest form, we spend our first year with our body finding out how to communicate with other people and their bodies. In all honesty, when babies come to the earth they already have the spiritual communication part down. That part comes more naturally to us than we want to admit.

We spend the first year as a baby looking at our fingers and sucking on our toes, while our organs are doing what they are created to do. Everything has its function, and that function is to help us stay alive and grow. Without having to think about it, our hearts beat, our lungs expand, and our organs do their job. This is the biggest blessing, but it also creates the biggest challenge: being mindful of our bodies. We have a role in supporting those organs.

Then we grow to be toddlers and learn how our legs work. We start to learn *independence*—finding out who we are and what our body can do on earth. This is where the separation starts to happen. We start to receive our own image from outside sources and from the feedback of our eyes. Our concept of who we are is often described by what the world and people around us say about us. What if we were to teach our children to continue to look inside—not outside—for that confirmation of who they are? What if we looked inside and asked questions to really find out the truth about our image? I find, in my practice and with myself, that this stage in life is where the body and mind deviate from the Spirit. As a result, we start to take on the natural man, which becomes a dominant force in driving our actions and behaviors.

STEP TO THE MARK

Elder Russell M. Nelson of the Quorum of the Twelve Apostles said, "Even that first look in the mirror can be more enjoyable *knowing we are created in his image.*"[4] So let's step to the first and fundamental mark that will set you on the path to becoming physically *fit for good*. If possible, walk to the nearest mirror. If this is not possible, commit now to act upon the following invitation soon.

Now remember, you should use this mirror to help you "step to the mark," not tempt you to "look beyond the mark" by leading you to either worship or loathe your physical features. This mirror should be used as an *instrument of reflection* so that you might learn to see and receive the image and glory of God (see 2 Corinthians 3:18).

Receive the Measure of Your Creation

Are you standing in front of a mirror? Yes? Great! No? Please get up, act upon the elements of your body, and place yourself in front of a mirror. Now look at yourself in the mirror for a few minutes, not moments. This will feel awkward at first. Take heed to ignore the negative or prideful thoughts that come so quickly when looking in a mirror. Notice your physical features. Watch as your eyes blink and as your chest slightly expands with each breath you take. Now move your arms and hands while pondering on the "thou art" doctrines given to Moses on that exceedingly high mountain. You are looking at a spiritual child of God who has a physical body created in the similitude of His Only Begotten. Receive the image of God by seeing your image in the mirror, your physical body as God sees it—the measure of your creation to become like Him. Remember, "when we look upon the human face we look upon the image of our Father and God; there is a divinity in each person, male and female, there is the heavenly, there is the divine."[5] Now be still and listen to the Spirit. Then record below what the Spirit speaks to you in thoughts or feelings about your body.

_____

_____

_____

_____

_____

_____

_____

_____

_____

_____

_____

Throughout the book, I recommend doing this mirror exercise often. This can be a moment of not only reflection of what you see in the mirror, but also a reflection of what you believe to be your truth so far in this life. This is one of my favorite exercises because it gives us the opportunity to ask some of my core life transformation questions: Is this true? Where did I learn this? How does it measure against the truth I've received from God? How can I start to combine these two reflections to become as one?

We can start to divide out the passions and temptations of the adversary. We can diligently strive to keep receiving His image. And remember who you are physically. You *are* a child of God. You can, and do, become physically connected to Jesus Christ when you take the sacrament each week. You can recommit when you look at your hands. You have a spirit, and it is controlling the elements of the body. You can ask yourself, what am I going to do with these hands? How can I best use these feet? How can I use these lips to speak kindness? And how can I use my eyes to see the reflection of myself and my brothers and sisters as they really are, as sons of daughters of God?

When you act upon this knowledge, the principles behind it can change your whole outlook on life and your experience here on earth. You can start to recognize that everyone is doing his or her best. If you are struggling because your best, or the best of someone else, doesn't seem to be reaching the mark, accept that as feedback from the Spirit that you have room to grow. Be willing to see how your capacity to act can be expanded. Be willing to work with gratitude to stretch into fulness of truth.

Your body is meant for you to experience joy—from the inside to the outside. The principles, patterns, and practices of fitness success will help you know the body is miraculous, and really start to believe it. Focus on the believing. Find out what is true to you. Be willing to do the exercise over and over. Each time, the reminder of who you are becomes clearer, and the lies of what the world tells you start to disappear.

Tips for the ultimate mirror exercise success:

- Pray first
- If you can't stand there for a few minutes, do a drive-by and say, "I am awesome."

Receive the Measure of Your Creation

- Take a moment to receive His image—even in the reflection of a car window or a puddle.

A young wife and mother of two children shared with me her experience with this activity. She was initially very resistant to attempt the exercise. She often avoided the mirrors in her home because they seemed to serve only as a tool to magnify her perceived physical imperfections, rather than as an instrument of reflection. In order to overcome this problem, she decided to kneel in prayer and ask for the strength to not "look beyond the mark," so that she might see herself physically as her Father in Heaven sees her. After her prayer, she faithfully stood in front of her mirror. She said, "It was as if a reverence came over me, and I felt grateful. I felt peaceful looking at the different parts of my body and thinking they are like God's. I then saw my body as a whole. It was beautiful to me. It was truly a gift from God!"

Your body is a gift from God! Your body is the most profound physical manifestation of your relationship to Him. It testifies that you are not far from Him. He has a resurrected "body of flesh and bones as tangible as [yours]" (D&C 130:22), meaning you have been blessed with a body of flesh and bones as tangible as His. You can receive His image. Believe that your body is the express image of God and is the greatest physical gift the Father has bestowed upon you thus far in your eternal progression. Your body is the measure of your creation. The measure of its natural shape, size, weight, age, or appearance has absolutely nothing to do with its true value. Your body has been measured as a temple of God given to you to become like Him (see 1 Corinthians 3:17).

"And God said, Let us make man in our image, after our likeness. . . . So God created man in his own image, in the image of God created he him; male and female created he them" (Genesis 1:26–27). Remember, how you *measure* your body, or in other words, how you view your body is the first mark that will set you on a path that will motivate you to become *fit for good*. Step to the mark and receive God's image. See your body as God sees it. Mark it as the measure of your creation—the physical evidence of your potential to become like Him.

Fit for Good

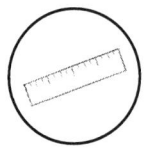 Receive God's image. Remember, your body is *the measure of your creation*—the physical manifestation of your potential to become like God.

CHAPTER 2

Yoke Yourself to the Power of Godliness

One beautiful, sunny Sunday afternoon, my family was visiting my wife's parents when, unexpectedly, our three-year-old daughter tore from her grandmother's arms and sprinted maliciously toward our one-year-old son, hitting him like a freight train. She drove him forcefully onto the living room floor and ripped a toy from his grasp while screaming, "That's mine!"

My wife and I looked at each other in disbelief as our son burst into tears. We had never seen our seemingly sweet little girl act with such aggression. My in-laws smiled at each other. It was time for me to forge my skills as a father. Rather than demonstrate my inexperience in public, I invited my daughter to go on a walk with me out to the back property. We found a dried creek bed and sat down in the soft sand to talk about what had happened. I began by reviewing the incident and asking my daughter *why* she had shoved her brother. To her it was obvious: he had "her" toy. Clamoring for what I might say next, I asked the one question that so many parents rely on to help guide their children: "What can we do to be more like Jesus?"

My daughter stopped sifting the sand and looked at me while squinting her eyes in concentration. She was earnestly pondering the question. I anticipated her answer, feeling confident that this three-year-old child would come to understand the error of her ways. I felt a sense of pride in my parenting skills. After a brief moment, her eyes brightened as she looked up at me. She had found the answer.

"Daddy, I know how," she said.

"How, sweetie?" I asked.

"You can grow a beard," she replied with excitement. "Then you would be more like Jesus!"

She threw me a mental curveball and caused me to chuckle. I gathered my thoughts and tried to clarify the question by focusing on how she could act more like the Savior, not how I could look more like Him. Eventually, we came to what I thought was a basic understanding of how she should treat her brother in the future, and we returned home. During the next few days, her "you can grow a beard" comment began to sink into my heart. In time, I realized I had been taught a powerful doctrine by her sweet innocence (see Alma 32:23).

YOKED

Let's leave the sandy creek bed in Arizona and return to the exceedingly high mountain with Moses to understand the doctrine my daughter had taught me. After learning his spiritual and physical identity and casting Satan out, Moses called upon God and saw His glory. The Father then revealed to Moses, like my daughter did to me, *how* to fill the measure of his creation. The Lord said, "Lo, I am with thee, even unto the end of thy days; for thou shalt deliver my people from bondage, even Israel my chosen" (Moses 1:26). This was the work the Lord had for Moses to do—to live in similitude of God's Only Begotten by serving the people of Israel as their physical savior.

Moses did much more than grow a beard in order to live in similitude of Christ. Consider a few of the following significant works that marked his life:

- He lived as a son of royalty (Exodus 2:10).
- He left his exalted state (Exodus 2:15).

Yoke Yourself to the Power of Godliness

- He became a shepherd to his Father's flock (Exodus 3:1).
- He performed mighty miracles (Exodus 8–13).
- He delivered his people from bondage (Exodus 13).
- He delivered his people from death (Exodus 14).
- He brought his family home to their promised land (Deuteronomy 34).
- He was taken up into heaven (Alma 45:19).

Can you see the *connection* between the actions that Moses performed and the actions that Christ would later perform? Moses's work was to *physically* live his life in similitude of Jesus Christ. Remember, you are of the same measured creation as Moses and have been called to *the same work*—to live in the similitude of God's Only Begotten. Now, we know that living in similitude of our perfect Savior is perfectly impossible unless we step to the mark by *connecting* ourselves to the enabling power of the second eternal mark—the *yoke* of Christ.

A yoke is a wooden crossbeam that is fastened over the shoulders of two animals to allow them to pull together the burden attached to them. A yoke has the capacity to physically make two animals that may or may not be equal in strength become *one*. Elder David A. Bednar of the Quorum of the Twelve has taught that "making and keeping sacred covenants yokes us to and with the Lord Jesus Christ."[1] We find these sacred covenants in the ordinances of the priesthood—the ordained outward, physical expressions of our inner commitments to follow the Savior: the first being the ordinance of baptism.

With baptism, we are physically immersed as an outward expression that we will take upon ourselves the name of Christ. One of the promises we make is to be "*willing* to bear one another's burdens, that they may be light" (Mosiah 18:8; emphasis added). Notice the word "willing" in that promise. When considered in all honesty, we as mortal beings have difficulty bearing our own burdens, let alone another's burdens. However, when we remain true to our baptismal covenant, we take upon ourselves the yoke of Christ that will allow the power of godliness to be manifest in our lives (see D&C 84:20).

The power of godliness will enable us to live *physically* in similitude of Him. That power *physically enabled* David to become a savior for the house of Israel with the sling of one smooth stone (see 1 Samuel 17). That power *physically* protected and *enabled* two thousand young men to save their Nephite brothers and sisters while defeating multiple Lamanite armies (see Alma 53–58). That power *physically enabled* Ammon to protect the king's flocks and become a savior for the king's servants and eventually for the king (see Alma 17–18). That power *physically enabled* the early pioneers to walk the plains and climb the Rocky Mountains to redeem Zion. The Savior's yoke—the power of godliness—will *physically enable* you to become *fit for good*.

Knowing what we are pulling for when we take upon ourselves the yoke of Christ can help motivate us. We gain a glimpse of it from Moses's questioning of the Father. "Moses called upon God, saying: Tell me, I pray thee, *why* these things are so? . . . And the Lord God said unto Moses: For mine own purpose have I made these things. Here is wisdom and it remaineth in me" (Moses 1:30–31; emphasis added). Moses, like any normal, inquisitive child would, asked the Father again, saying, "Be merciful unto thy servant, O God, and tell me concerning this earth, and the inhabitants thereof, and also the heavens, and then thy servant will be content" (Moses 1:36). Surely pleased with His son's desire to know more, the Lord then revealed to Moses the purpose of His work, saying, "For behold, this is my work and glory—to bring to pass the immortality and eternal life of man" (Moses 1:39).

Now let's follow Moses's example and continue in the role of an inquisitive child by asking again the question: *why* does Heavenly Father want to bring to pass the immortality and eternal life of man? The prophet Lehi provided the answer, saying, "Adam fell that man might be; and men are, that they might have joy" (2 Nephi 2:25). President David O. McKay further confirmed this truth by explaining that "happiness is the purpose and design of existence."[2]

Let this doctrine settle on your mind for a moment. The answer to why God created you and me is to have joy! The purpose of your

Yoke Yourself to the Power of Godliness

soul—meaning your spirit and body (see D&C 88:15)—in this life and in the next is to be at one, or yoked, with Christ so you can experience a *fulness* of joy and happiness (see D&C 93:33). Take a few moments, and use the lines below to write down how this doctrine makes you feel. Remember, when we take upon ourselves the yoke of Christ, the power of godliness is manifest in our lives. That power enables us to act, rather than be acted upon, in the only way (see John 14:6) that can fill the measure of our creation with a fulness of joy.

_____

_____

_____

_____

_____

_____

_____

_____

_____

_____

_____

_____

_____

_____

_____

_____

_____

From the moment we left the physical warmth, protection, and provision of our mother's womb, we have been acting to fulfill this purpose—experiencing a fulness of joy and happiness. The fallen elements of this cold and dreary world we were born into *acted upon us*, causing us to reflexively cry out. Our cry caused our mothers to draw close to us. We became yoked to her calming voice, familiar heartbeat, and sweet nourishment. This connection filled our fragile frame with a measure of joy. Within moments, the opposition of this fallen world *acted upon us* again in the form of a growing hunger or some other physical agitation. Again, our bodies reflexively cried out, yoking us to those that would help us fill the measure of our creation with a measure of joy.

We repeated this process over and over for several weeks. Then, it happened—the moment we became more like our Father in Heaven than we had ever been before. Our spirits, not the environment or our inherent reflexes, *acted upon* the elements of our body (see 2 Nephi 2:14). It was a conscious smile, a cry, or a reach of an arm—a movement meant to fill the measure of our creation with happiness. From that moment, we began to act upon the elements of our bodies in an effort to gain greater dominion over them so that we could experience a "greater happiness" (Abraham 1:2). We endured thousands of bumps, bruises, and bad days learning how to physically reach, roll, crawl, walk, and run, in an effort to yoke ourselves to that which would fill the measure of our creation with more joy.

STEP TO THE MARK

There were once two young orphan brothers that were purchased from a slave trader by a master architect. The young boys were blessed in the home of their master as he provided them with shelter, protection, and love. The two boys began to learn from and about their master as he created the most magnificent mansions. The brothers worked side by side with their master and grew into skilled architects themselves.

One day, the master shared with the boys the news that they had been commissioned by the king to construct two magnificent mansions for his

Yoke Yourself to the Power of Godliness

family. The king required that the mansions be built with only the best materials and techniques available. They were to last forever. The master architect informed the boys that the king would provide all the materials necessary to build the mansions and had already paid their commission in full. Their master then provided them with the architectural plans for each mansion and informed them that he would be gone for several seasons, giving each brother a stewardship over the construction of one of the mansions.

The master architect left his apprentices with his blessing, and with excitement and great determination, the young apprentices began their work. Day after day, month after month, they labored, and the mansions began to take shape. Both apprentices were blessed by their work. They found great joy in their work. In time, the younger apprentice began to notice that the money, though sufficient, was diminishing faster than anticipated. He felt that the cost of furnishing the finest materials and the time he was spending was cutting too deep into his profit. He began to use slightly less than the best materials and methods. He cut corners in places that would not lessen the appearance of the mansion, and that increased his free time. By doing this, the younger apprentice saw his profit margin, as well as his social status, substantially increase.

The older apprentice remained true to his master's plan. From the footings to the finish, he built the king's mansion day after day as if his master were at his side. In time, the boys finished their mansions, and the king came in great majesty with his royal courts to claim the mansions for his family. The king visually inspected both mansions; their appearances were magnificent! Both apprentices were presented before the king. Their bows before the king brought them to their knees in shock as the saw the familiar face of their master under the crown. Their master and king praised both for their work, and then handed them each the deed and the key to the mansion they had built. Inscribed upon each key were the words, "Forever Yours, My Son."

What was the difference between the two apprentices? The elder apprentice had chosen to remain yoked to the master in his work while the younger one had not. Both had received their physical mansion, the measure of their creation; however, the joy they would experience therein would vary. One would rest in peace knowing that his mansion would last forever; the other would not.

Let's compare the building of these mansions to the building of our bodies. What are we yoked to when we exercise? When we exercise, do we do so yoked primarily to the fading particle of joy that comes when others notice the newly contoured shape of our body? Do we exercise yoked to a measure of pleasure that comes when we finally shed those extra pounds or complete a sub-sixty-minute 10 km race? Do we exercise yoked to the panacea of peace that comes when our exercise efforts help us fend off a pending heart attack, stroke, or diabetes? Exercising while yoked to these things will provide us with a "moment" or "measure" of joy; however, the joy these moments mete will fail to fill the measure of our creation with a *fulness* of joy.

Only by taking upon yourself the yoke of Christ can you have the capacity to fill the measure of your creation with a fulness of joy. His yoke was hewn for you and me in the Garden of Gethsemane. It has the power to pull us and help us pull each other through any experience in this life, no matter the magnitude. His yoke pulls for us so we might have *eternal* joy—the joy that is "most joyous to the soul" (1 Nephi 11:23). Remember, Christ's yoke has the power to bless us "in all things, both *temporal* and spiritual" (Mosiah 2:41; emphasis added), including in our efforts to exercise dominion over the elements of our bodies to get physically *fit for good*.

Here's how you can yoke yourself to Christ as you exercise. Please list below what you value most in your life.

1. _____
2. _____
3. _____
4. _____
5. _____

Yoke Yourself to the Power of Godliness

I can't read what you have listed, but I am confident that at least one item on your list has something to do with your relationships. You value your relationships with those whom you love; the *same thing* our Father in Heaven values.

There are many ways that our Father shows us that we are of value to Him; however, nothing witnesses our value to Him more than when He gave us "his only begotten Son, that whosoever believeth in him should not perish, but have everlasting life" (John 3:16). In turn, Christ showed how much He values us when He suffered for us in the garden and upon the cross. He has invited you to do the same, to "take [His] yoke upon you" (Matthew 11:29), and to pull with Him to experience the fulness of joy that comes from blessing the lives of others. This invitation is not limited to your work in church, in your profession, or in your home; it also includes the work you do when you physically exercise.

When you focus your fitness efforts on increasing your physical capacity to give of yourself in similitude of Christ, you will be "exercise-yoked to Christ." Take, for example, the young father of four who decides to ride his bike to work each day. He has no difficulty on the way to work, as the path to his work is a series of small hills, with one extended, steep hill that he enjoys riding downhill right to his office door. However, each day after work he dreads that extended uphill ride, as it becomes a lung-busting and leg-burning battle toward home. Week after week, he struggles up the hill, stopping every few hundred feet to catch his breath and question why he is doing this. He first answers, *to get fit.*

He then asks the question "why" again, this time to sharpen his focus and step to the mark. *Not just to lose weight or to lower my cholesterol,* he thinks, *but to increase my physical capacity to be like Christ for my wife and my children.* With that thought, he works his way up the mammoth hill, pulling with Christ (figuratively growing a beard for his wife and children), while filling the measure of his creation with joy.

Step to the mark by exercising while being yoked to Christ. When your fitness efforts are focused on increasing your physical capacity to live in similitude of Christ in behalf of those you love, your fitness efforts will not fail because you will be yoked to the One that will enable you to become physically *fit for good*.

This principle and process of yoking yourself to Christ will not change as circumstances change. How we apply this process may vary, but the principle, pattern, and practice always stay the same. I love that about our Heavenly Father. In a world of inconsistency, He sets patterns to help guide us and make things easier. Once you learn the principle, you get to practice the pattern and learn precept upon precept.

In 2007, I was floundering for anything consistent. I had just had my fourth child, my husband had gone to basic training for the army, I had sold our franchise, and I had moved with my kids, waiting to find out where the Lord would send me. I was overweight at this time in my life, but as I have found in the recent years after my weigh loss, it had nothing to do with my weight. I needed something solid to yoke myself to. That year was the first time I actively put this principle to the test in my own life. To my surprise, it led to fitness success. I lost eighty pounds that year, but I found something even more miraculous; I found Christ and the fulness of joy that comes when I yoke my efforts to His. I found boundless energy. Even with my husband deployed for sixteen months and absent for two years, and even with raising small kids, learning this principle and following these patterns set me up for success *every day*!

In the past ten years, I have lived in five states and overseas in another country. I have lived six of those years raising my kids by myself while my husband served our country. I haven't lived by my family in over two decades. I have had no lack of opportunity to feel alone. I have had no lack of hardship. I have only experienced ease when I lean into these principles and walk with faith.

It is a choice you can make everyday. I know from the last ten years of working with sisters that every situation is unique. How you will apply these principles will be specific to your own situation, but the outcome can be the same for you. You can feel joy. You can have fitness success while exercising these patterns in your life.

Yoke Yourself to the Power of Godliness

Here are my top three tips to yoke yourself to Christ and make things simple as you become physically *fit for good*:

1. Stop floundering and decide. Step over the line and decide to yoke yourself to Christ. Choose to let go of the world and walk in faith with Him.

2. Recognize the pattern. Practice every day to become consistent in living these principles, like our Heavenly Father.

3. Ask yourself these questions:

   - What can I do today to yoke myself to Christ?
   - How does this help me feel joy?
   - How am I making the physical connection today to become more like my Savior?
   - How can I teach this principle and show these patterns to those I love?

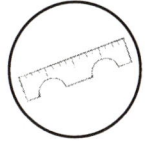

Yoke yourself to Christ when you exercise. Remember, *His yoke will enable* the measure of your creation to be filled with a fulness of joy.

Fit for Good

LINE UPON LINE SUMMARIES

On Your Marks

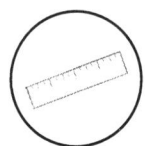

Receive God's image. Remember, your body is *the measure of your creation*—the physical manifestation of your potential to become like God.

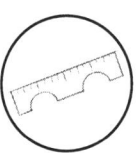

Yoke yourself to Christ when you exercise. Remember, *His yoke will enable* the measure of your creation to be filled with a fulness of joy.

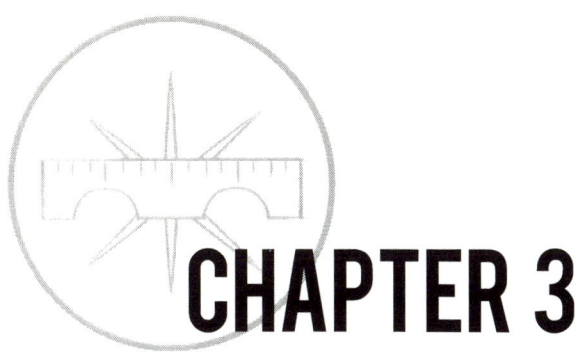

CHAPTER 3

Consecrate to Be Quickened

We decided to climb it because it was there. My family had just moved to La Verkin, Utah, at the base of the small mountain ridge. Every summer morning since our arrival, my two older brothers and I, ages nine, eight, and six, stared at that mountain ridge as it called for us to conquer it. Early one morning, before Mom and Dad could ask where we were going, we decided to answer the call. My oldest brother Rob led the way as we worked our way through the neighborhood to the base of the ridge. We found a trailhead and started our ascent to the top, throwing rocks and chasing lizards along the way.

The trail eventually came to an end at the base of what, through the eyes of a six-year-old boy, looked like a massive cliff. Without hesitation, Rob, who was part mountain goat, traversed up the cliff with little difficulty. Now, as the youngest of the three boys, I took every opportunity to prove myself, so I set off to climb the small cliff before my brother Corban could. The higher I climbed, the faster my confidence fell until, just a few feet from the top, I discontinued all efforts to move. I clung to the cliff face as I forcefully testified to my brothers that I was going to die. Rob reached down from the top and encouraged me to grab his hand. I refused, knowing quite well in my mature six-year-old mind that if I let go of my grip on the cliff, I would plummet a tragic eight feet to my definite death. My brother Corban quickly came to my rescue and climbed up to me. I found comfort in having him by my side until I saw the sheer terror on his face as he clung on and then quickly joined the testimony meeting of our upcoming deaths. Rob continued his efforts to encourage us to reach for his hand. Corban and I ignored him as we looked at each other, feeding off of our collective fear.

Suddenly, Corban stopped crying. I watched as his demeanor changed from sheer terror to absolute confidence. Corban looked at me and said, "We need to pray!" So, we did. Corban prayed, asking Heavenly Father to give us the strength to make it safely to the top. After the prayer, I felt a surge of strength and power. I reached up to grab Rob's hand as Corban supported me from below. Now, the higher I climbed, the more I felt the Spirit, and eventually I made it safely to the top. I crept onto my stomach and helped Rob pull Corban up. We stood up and turned to the east to see the rising sun coming up over the horizon. I remember feeling an overwhelming love from, and for, the Lord, having just experienced the physical salvation of His hand in our young lives. We turned back for home, *quickened* by a power that came through prayer.

QUICKENED

After you covenanted to take the yoke of Christ upon yourself through the ordinance of baptism, you received a gift—the gift of the Holy Ghost (see Acts 2:38). This spiritual gift was given to help guide, comfort, and quicken you in the yoke of Christ. Most of us are very familiar with the Holy Ghost's power to guide and comfort us; however, His power to *quicken*, the third eternal mark, is often overlooked.

Moses gained a powerful testimony of the quickening power of the Spirit that transfigured him on that exceedingly high mountain. After his initial face-to-face visit with the Father, Moses fell to the earth and remained there for several hours due to physical exhaustion. After recovering from his fatigue, he said, "Mine own eyes have beheld God; but not my natural, but my spiritual eyes, for my natural eyes could not have beheld; for I should have withered and died in his presence; but his glory

Consecrate to Be Quickened

was upon me; and I beheld his face, for I was transfigured before him" (Moses 1:11). Elder Bruce R. McConkie of the Quorum of the Twelve Apostles wrote the following about transfiguration: "Transfiguration is a special change in appearance and nature which is wrought upon a person or thing by the power of God. This divine transformation is from a lower to a higher state; it results in a more exalted, impressive, and glorious condition. . . . By the power of the Holy Ghost many prophets have been transfigured so as to stand in the presence of God and view the visions of eternity."[1]

This doctrine is confirmed in Doctrine and Covenants section 67, where we learn that transfiguration, the *physical transformation* from a lower to a higher state, comes by the power of the Holy Ghost: "for no man has seen God at any time in the *flesh*, except *quickened* by the Spirit of God" (D&C 67:11; emphasis added). The gospel definition of the word "quicken" is "to make alive, to resurrect, or to change a person so he [or she] can be in the presence of God."[2] From Moses's experience, we learn that quickening is a spiritual influence that has a physical effect.

Now here is a wonderful truth: we can experience a form of quickening (a physical transformation from a lower to a higher state) every day of our lives! This happens when we choose to act upon the elements of our body under the spiritual direction and influence of the Holy Ghost. Elder Parley P. Pratt described the quickening influence the Spirit has upon our bodies:

> The gift of the Holy Ghost . . . quickens all the intellectual faculties, increases, enlarges, expands and purifies all the natural passions and affections, and adapts them, by the gift of wisdom, to their lawful use. . . . It develops beauty of person, *form and features*. It tends to *health, vigor,* animation and social feeling. It invigorates all the faculties of the *physical* and intellectual man [and woman]. It *strengthens,* and gives tone to the *nerves.* In short, it is, as it were, *marrow to the bone,* joy to the heart, light to the eyes, music to the ears, and *life to the whole thing.*[3]

What a wonderful, spiritually induced physical transformation! We often see dramatic forms of this physical transformation in the lives of members of the Church. We see it in those that receive baptism and the gift of the Holy Ghost. We see it when a family member or friend leaves the temple endowed with power from on high. We see it when our young men and young women return from serving honorable missions. These individuals are those who have experienced a quickening of the Spirit as they have taken upon them the yoke of Christ, filling the measure of their creation with the light and joy of His countenance (see D&C 88:51–62).

We know that the Holy Ghost has a quickening effect upon our bodies. Can our physical health then have an effect on the Spirit's ability to quicken us? Elder Richard G. Scott of the Quorum of the Twelve Apostles declared that, "spiritual communication can be enhanced by good health practices."[4]

We know that "the spirit and the body together are the soul of man" (D&C 88:15), and that "what affects one affects the other."[5] By my own experience, I know this is true. When I fail to pay heed to my physical health, I find that my ability to *act* under the influence of the Spirit is limited, and I find myself often *reacting* more to the maladies of mortality. I become more inclined to lose my temper or to become more apathetic to my responsibilities. I become more fatigued and less likely to answer the call to serve. Spiritually, like Nephi lamented, I begin to "linger in the valley of sorrow" and physically let "my flesh waste away" and "my strength slacken" (2 Nephi 4:26). In essence, I begin to forfeit my capacity to experience the quickening companionship of the Holy Ghost.

Have you experienced that same phenomenon? Are your words to your family and friends often sharper when you're feeling physically dull? Do you find it hard to "succor the weak, lift up the hands which hang down, and strengthen the feeble knees" (D&C 81:5) of others when your own hands hang down and your knees seem ready to buckle because of physical weakness and fatigue?

We can limit this! When Nephi felt his strength slacken and his heart begin to weep because of his flesh, he declared, "Awake, my soul! No longer droop in sin. Rejoice, O my heart, and give place no more for the enemy of my soul" (2 Nephi 4:26–28). Nephi recognized that he needed to act in a manner that would expel the influence of the adversary in his

Consecrate to Be Quickened

life. He knew that he could call upon God and be "filled . . . with his love, even unto the consuming," or in other words, *quickening* "of [his] flesh" (2 Nephi 4:21). Like my brother did on our quickening cliff, Nephi cried unto the Lord for strength (see 2 Nephi 4:31–34). Nephi then concluded his psalm with these words—the key to the quickening influence of the Spirit: "I know that God will give liberally to him that asketh . . . not amiss" (2 Nephi 4:35). We know that regular exercise can strengthen us when our flesh begins to waste away; however, we often "ask amiss" in our exercise efforts by simply failing to ask.

STEP TO THE MARK

A mother once shared with me an "out of the mouth of babes" experience she had while potty training her two-year-old son (Psalm 8:2). For several weeks they had worked together, and her son was close to mastering the skill. On this particular day, she wanted to teach her son about privacy. She informed him that this time he would go to the bathroom by himself so that he could have some "privacy," and that she would be right outside the door to help if needed. She closed the door and waited. After a few moments, she heard her little boy's voice through the door.

"Mom?"

"Yes, Son?"

"Is Holy with me?"

"I'm sorry, Son. I don't know who Holy is."

"You know, Mom. Holy the Ghost. Is He with me when I have privacy?"

The mother smiled and replied, "Yes, Son. I'm sure Holy is with you."

Consider this child's innocent question. He wanted to know if the Holy Ghost could be with him no matter the setting. The answer is a definite yes! In fact, this is the blessing the Lord desires to bless us with each Sabbath day as we renew our baptismal covenants by partaking of the sacrament, "that they may always have his Spirit to be with them" (D&C 20:77).

Fit for Good

If the blessing of the sacrament is to have the Spirit with you *always*, ask yourself this question: Have you had the Spirit with you when you exercised? Have you ever invited Him? If we are not consistently inviting the Spirit to be with us as we exercise, we will eventually fail in our efforts to become physically *fit for good*.

Why? Because the Holy Ghost's quickening influence on your body is more powerful than any special fruit drink, vitamin pack, or training program you can consume or participate in. He is more than a personal trainer. He is the personal transformer that Heavenly Father has sent to transform and quicken us from a lower to a higher physical state—a *fit for good* celestial state (see D&C 88:28–29).

Think about how you can invite the Spirit to be with you when you exercise. Praying for the Spirit is an excellent start. Other ways to invite the Spirit may include remembering to yoke yourself to Christ as you begin your yoga class, dressing in modest exercise attire, or refraining from arguing with your teenage son the morning before you exercise. Record your thoughts below.

_____

_____

_____

_____

_____

_____

_____

_____

_____

_____

_____

_____

Consecrate to Be Quickened

Remember the father in the last chapter who rode his bike up that monstrous hill home from work each day? What might happen in his effort to climb that hill if he chose to pray with real intent for the companionship of the Spirit to be with him as he peddled? That hill could become an "exceedingly high mountain" for him—a hill that could help yoke him to Christ as he exercises to increase his physical fitness to bless the lives of his family. With the quickening power of the Spirit present, each push up the hill would transform this father from a lower to a higher physical state, a state that would *increase his physical capacity* to live in the similitude of the Only Begotten.

Think for a moment how inviting the Spirit to join you in your workout would change your exercise experience. Would your focus change? Would you find more motivation to reach your fitness goals? Would you find more joy in your exercise efforts? You and I both know the answer to each of these questions is a firm and fit yes!

So, step to the third eternal mark—just like you pray over the food you eat to "nourish and strengthen your body" at each meal, commit to pray for the companionship of the Spirit to be with you as you exercise. In your prayer, "consecrate thy [exercise] performance unto thee, that thy [exercise] performance may be for the welfare of thy soul" (2 Nephi 32:9). As you invite the Spirit to be with you as you exercise, His presence will *quicken* you physically. He will *quicken* all your "natural passions and affections" and adapt them, "by the gift of wisdom, to their lawful use," into a state that will develop the beauty of your person in "form and features;" a state that will bless your body with "health, vigor, animation and social feeling;" a state that will quicken "all the faculties" of your "physical and intellectual man." "In short," a state that will give "marrow to [your] bone[s], joy to [your] heart, light to [your] eyes, music to [your] ears, and *life to [your] whole being.*"[6]

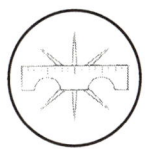

Invite the Spirit to be with you when you exercise. Remember, *His power will quicken* the measure of your creation so you can experience a fulness of joy.

LINE UPON LINE SUMMARY

On Your Marks

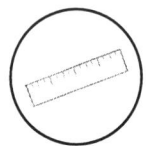

Receive God's image. Remember, your body is *the measure of your creation*—the physical manifestation of your potential to become like God.

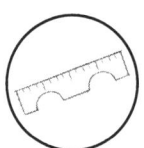

Yoke yourself to Christ when you exercise. Remember, *His yoke will enable* the measure of your creation to be filled with a fulness of joy.

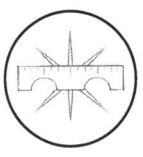

Invite the Spirit to be with you when you exercise. Remember, *His power will quicken* the measure of your creation so you can experience a fulness of joy.

PART TWO
Get Set

After stepping to the starting mark, the runners were given the command to "Get Set!" With this command, each runner in the boot race crouched down, dug their boots into the asphalt, and held their breath. Why? To act upon the elements of their body and to prepare for the opposition of every asphalt-pounding step they would take toward the finish line. This opposition would serve as a blessing to those who had the physical capacity to properly act upon the elements of their body. It would become a painful curse of road rash and broken bones for those who did not. Part two will help you get set for the sweat, the fiery darts, and the experimentation that will increase, resist, and teach you how to get *fit for good*.

CHAPTER 4

By the Sweat of Your Brow

Our father spoke with authority and bestowed upon us these loving *words of wisdom*. "Boys," he said, "you will not step one foot onto the pond. If you do go on the ice and it breaks, you could die."

We each gulped and nodded our heads in the affirmative. Judging by the raised eyebrows and questioning look on our father's face, it was obvious that our nods were not enough. Not wanting to jeopardize our chance to sled down the massive hill next to the pond, my oldest brother, Rob, spoke up. "Yes, Dad. We will stay off the pond."

Satisfied with Rob's acceptance of the responsibility, he bestowed his blessing. Rob, now twelve years of age; Corban, ten; and I, nine, quickly donned our snow gear and headed out the door to make the most of the nearly two feet of white *wilderness* that had fallen in Prescott, Arizona, and given us a rare gift—a snow day away from school.

The sledding hill was located next to the pond on our grandfather's small ranch in the foothills. We hiked from our house to the ranch, dragging our sleds behind us while our family dog, Chewbacca, crisscrossed along our path, sniffing out jackrabbits and quail. By the time we arrived, the temperature had risen, making the snow perfect for sledding. Rob marked out the line for our path, and then Corban took the virgin run down the steep hill. With the path now outlined, we got to work building up the run's brims and banks to ensure a fast and thrill-filled ride.

For the next hour, we sailed down the hill and ran back up over and over again. In time, and according to our genetic makeup as rambunctious boys, we began to grow tired of sledding. We focused our efforts on building a snow cave while trying to distract ourselves from the pond that beckoned us to explore its ice-covered beauty. While digging through the snow, one of us happened upon a stick and in line with his genetic makeup, threw it on the middle of his suppressed obsession—the pond. Reflexively, Chewbacca acted according to his genetic makeup as a dog and headed for the pond to fetch the stick. All three of our young hearts sunk as we saw our beloved ball of white fur scamper out onto the pond. Each of us screamed, "Chewbacca, stop!"

For a moment, he stopped and turned to look at us, seemingly confused by our commands. We all paused, breathlessly wondering if the ice would hold. He then scampered the remaining few feet, fetched the stick and came to us. We smothered him with hugs, and then scolded the one who had thrown the stick. To this day, my brothers and I still debate whom that person was. However, our active and pond-focused minds quickly realized that Chewbacca had safely traversed the pond's plate of ice.

Digging deep into our shallow logic, we concluded that Dad had made a decision to restrict our freedom to play on the iced-over pond without the knowledge that the ice was strong enough to hold Chewbacca and, therefore, us. To further establish the evidence in our favor, we began to test the strength of the ice covering the pond. We dug through the snow, pried some large rocks from the cold ground, and then hurled them onto the pond. They bounced off the ice and made a pinging sound that echoed up the canyon. With each rock we launched onto the ice, the more our confidence grew that the ice could hold us. So Corban and I began to play a little of game of chicken. Corban shuffled a few feet from the bank onto the ice and came back. I followed suit and crept out in my moon boots just a few feet farther than Corban had. Rob suggested we stop, remembering his responsibility. However, it was too late. Corban had already begun to run down from the hill, throwing himself tummy-first onto the ice. He slid, spun, and screamed in delight, slowly coming to a stop near the middle of the pond. "Beat that!" he shouted triumphantly, as he struggled to get to his feet on the ice. When he did, we heard a sound that stopped time.

Crack! The ice began to break. Corban dropped down onto his hands and knees trying to disperse his body weight, but it was too late. The ice opened up and began to slowly swallow him. I stood frozen in fear as I watched Corban cling to the icy edge and plead for help. Rob's Boy Scout life-saving skills kicked in. "Human chain! Human chain! We need to make a human chain!" yelled Rob frantically. He dropped down onto his stomach and instructed me to get on my stomach and crawl behind him, holding onto his ankles. We carefully made our way out to Corban. Rob tried to pull him up over the edge of the ice. The combined force of our weight was too great for the ice. It started to crack under Rob and continued to separate under me. All three of us fell forward into the frigid and unforgiving pond. I instinctively pushed off Rob to get to the surface. I struggled to anchor myself on the edge of the ice and began to scream for help. Corban and Rob both surfaced and thrashed in the water in an effort to fend off our seemingly certain death. Quickly, my brothers joined me in what I thought was a united shout for survival; however, I soon realized they were screaming not for help, but for me to stand up!

I cautiously let go of the ice's edge and let myself sink into the pond. My feet found the bottom as the water line serendipitously settled just below the level of my chin. A sudden rush of comfort and joy shot through my shivering body because I thought that I might live another day. My brothers waded past me and began to break a path with their elbows through the ice as their teeth chattered from the ice water that was now biting at their bones. We eventually made it to shore, gathered our sleds, and trudged solemnly up the hill to seek refuge in grandma's house. With each soaked and chill-filled step, our father's words of wisdom ran through our minds as we discussed how we would "break" the news to him.

SWEAT

My brothers and I were not the first children to face their father after disobeying his words of wisdom. In the Garden of Eden, our Father in Heaven gave Adam and Eve these words of wisdom: "But of the tree of the knowledge of good and evil, thou shalt not eat of it, nevertheless, thou mayest choose for thyself, for it is given unto thee; but, remember that I forbid it, for in the day thou eatest thereof thou shalt surely die" (Moses 3:17). Like the Father's Word of Wisdom given in section 89 of the Doctrine and Covenants, this word of wisdom was also given to Adam and Eve for their temporal salvation; it was a "principle with a promise" (D&C 89:3). The promise was that they would have continual "health in the navel and marrow to their bones" (D&C 89:18), or in other words, immortality as long as they did not partake of the fruit of the tree of knowledge of good and evil.

In time, Adam and Eve chose to transgress God's command and partake of the forbidden fruit. Their choice came with a consequence. They become mortal and were cast out of the beautiful Garden of Eden. They were introduced into the "wilderness," a fallen world that would constantly oppose them and eventually overcome them in death, returning the elements of their bodies back to the dust from which they were formed (Moses 4:25). However, just like my father did before my brothers and I entered our white wilderness of snow, the Father gave Adam and Eve further words of wisdom before they entered the wilderness of this fallen world. He said unto them, "By the *sweat* of thy face shalt thou eat *bread*, until thou shalt return unto the ground" (Moses 4:25; emphasis added).

We know that the Lord's words of wisdom are given by our Father "for a principle with promise" (D&C 89:3). What is the promise associated with the principle of sweat by labor (see Moses 5:1)? We can learn of this promise by better understanding the sweat that is associated with it. There are three things that can cause us to sweat: temperature, disease, and physical exertion. Each one of these factors is a derivative of the wilderness of our fallen world. The first two cause sweat to form on our brows when the elements of our bodies are *acted upon by the wilderness*.

By the Sweat of Your Brow

The last causes us to sweat when *we act upon* the elements of our bodies against the opposition of the fallen world which we live in. This type of sweat will bead on our brows with a promise—the promise to "eat bread."

In scripture, "bread" symbolizes much more than just a combination of flour, water, sugar, and salt. It is the product of man's dominion over the elements that when partaken of can delay death and provide man with the energy to act rather than to be acted upon. However, the full blessings and benefits of eating bread are only experienced when it is coupled with the sweat of physical exertion, the manifestation of our acting upon the elements of our bodies against the opposition of the wilderness that is found in our fallen world.

The wilderness of our fallen world is essential. After our Savior was baptized, He was "led up of the Spirit into the *wilderness*" to commune with God (Joseph Smith Translation Matthew 4:1 [in Matthew 4:1, footnote *b*]; emphasis added). Now why did the Spirit lead Christ into the wilderness to commune with God? Why not to His home or the synagogue? Elder James E. Talmage answered this question, saying that the Savior retired to the wilderness to fast with a primary purpose, so "that His mortal body might the more completely be subjected to His divine spirit."[1]

Ponder on Elder Talmage's words—so "that [Christ's] mortal body might the more completely be subjected to His divine spirit." What a powerful principle. The wilderness coupled with His fast provided Him the opportunity to gain greater dominion over the elements of His body. This dominion was vital to the Father's plan of salvation, for it was the sweat of Christ's brow in His wilderness experience that blessed Him with *the increased physical capacity to act* upon the fallen elements of His body, that He might bear the future burden that would cause Him to sweat drops of blood in our behalf in the Garden of Gethsemane.

You too can claim the same promise. You can increase your physical capacity to act by sweating in the wilderness. You don't have to travel to the nearest national park to find wilderness. You can find it in your living room, down the street, up a flight of stairs, or in the gym. It is the "wilderness of opposition" that will come when you exercise. Exercise is a mini wilderness of opposition that will cause your brow to bead with sweat as you act to "more completely" subject the fallen elements of your body to your divine spirit. Exercise will cause your respiration rate, heart rate, and body temperature to rise. The elements of your body will strongly plead for you to stop; however, if you continue to exercise dominion over your body, sweat will form on your brow, and in time, the elements of your body will obey. Their obedience will increase your physical capacity to act in a manner that will fill the measure of your creation with joy.

GET SET

I loved school field trips as a child. They served as mini vacations from the monotony of school. I vividly remember one such vacation. My third grade class visited the local pioneer museum. The museum director had prepared various activities to give us the opportunity to physically experience the late eighteenth century. The director of the museum sat us down on the grass and described what the activities would be. She explained that we would be divided into groups and that each group would get to do an activity. She proceeded to show us some fabric for quilting and a long string that would be used to make a wax candle. The next item she held up sent a chill of excitement up and down my spine. "One group will use whittling knives to make a wooden pioneer spoon," she said.

I could hardly keep myself still. My body fidgeted in happy anticipation at the thought of playing with knives. I am confident that my teacher was aware of this and wisely placed me in the group that would be making wax candles. I protested as best I could. I finally accepted my assignment, and with depressed shoulders and one very prominent lower lip, I followed my classmates to the wax-candle area. The volunteer stationed there introduced herself and began to describe the candle-making process. My facial expression quickly changed from deep disappointment to utter despair. Rather than wielding a knife to create a masterpiece, I was going to spend the next twenty minutes walking in

By the Sweat of Your Brow

endless circles dipping a string into a bucket of cold water and then into hot wax. I couldn't believe it. I was having a nightmare. The volunteer, with a smile and a kind invitation to be patient, handed us each a string. We began our journey, dipping our strings in a barrel of cold water and then in a barrel of hot wax over and over and over again.

I glanced over at the whittlers. They seemed to be having the time of their lives. Their wood shavings flew through the air with each stroke of their sharp knives. I continued to circle and dip my string in the bucket of water and then the bucket of wax again and again, hoping to be rescued from this wilderness of waxing.

My despair was broken by the volunteer's words. "Keep dipping," she said. "Something magical will happen soon." Around and around we went. After each dip, I examined my string. Nothing. *This is not working*, I thought to myself. *I wish I was whittling*! Around we continued.

Suddenly, one of my classmates squealed with excitement. "Look!" she said, as she held up her string. There was a small but definitely visible accumulation of wax on her wick.

At that moment, something awakened within me. Maybe there *is* something to the endless circles and dipping. My focus shifted ever so slightly from whittling to waxing. My pain and frustration lessened with each dip as I anticipated the fruit of my efforts. Our kind volunteer continued to encourage us. "The wax is building up. Your candle will grow bigger and bigger with each dip. Good work! The rest of you, keep dipping. Don't give up!" she said.

Around we went, again and again. Periodically, one of my classmates shouted out with excitement when their candle started to take form. In time, my candle began to form. At that moment, I felt a small jolt of joy. In fact, my joy increased with each subsequent dip as I watched my candle grow larger and larger. Now my focus completely shifted from whittling to waxing. I was determined to make the biggest candle I could. I broke free from the circling line and ran back and forth between the two barrels dipping my wick as fast as I could. The volunteer quickly corralled me and gently informed me that if I dipped my candle too fast, it would fail to properly form and eventually slough off my wick. However, if I was consistent in my dipping and followed the guidelines she had set, my candle would form with a solid and sound shape. With this new understanding, I found my place in line and continued to dip my candle. Each purposeful, consistent, and controlled dip helped the candle grow larger. Whittling was the furthest thing from my mind. I spent every last second of the field trip dipping my candle into the water and wax to increase my candle's capacity to fill the measure of its creation (see 3 Nephi 12:14–16).

Regular physical exercise is like the waxing of a candle. At times it will feel like the elements of your body are "[combining] to hedge up [your] way." So when your exercise efforts cause your brow to sweat, wipe it off and welcome the wilderness of physical exercise that "shall give thee experience, and shall be for thy good" (D&C 122:7). With each dip into the wilderness of exercise, you will sweat, and thus claim the Father's promise of increased physical capacity to act upon the elements of this world to fill the measure of your creation with joy.

Remember, at one point in my dipping I lost focus and broke free from the line to dip faster and faster. Had I continued at such a pace, my candle would have failed to form properly. The same goes for the physical formation of your body. Always ensure that you are safe *to* exercise and safe *when* you exercise. The Lord has counseled us "that all these things are done in wisdom and order; for it is not requisite that a man should run faster than he has strength. And again, it is expedient that he should be diligent, that thereby he might win the prize; therefore, all things must be done in order" (Mosiah 4:27).

Take a moment and write down how you can ensure that you are safe to exercise and safe when you exercise. Here a few questions to consider. Have I had a physical in the last year? Do I wear the proper protective gear when I exercise? Do my family members know where I am when I exercise?

By the Sweat of Your Brow

_____
_____
_____
_____
_____
_____
_____
_____
_____

Get set for the sweat of physical exercise by remembering our Father's words of wisdom: "By the sweat of thy face" (*physical exercise*) "shalt thou eat bread" (*live*) (Moses 4:25). Just as my earthy father's words of wisdom were meant to save his children's lives, our Heavenly Father's words of wisdom are meant to give His children life. Claim the promise of this principle by welcoming the wilderness of physical exercise. Remember that with each episode of brow-sweating exercise, you are figuratively "dipping" your body into the "hot wax" of physical exertion that will bless you with "health in [your] navel and marrow to [your] bones" (D&C 89:18) that *will increase your physical capacity to act* and fill the measure of your creation with joy.

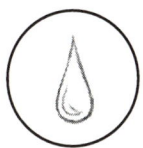

Sweat in the wilderness of regular exercise. The *sweat of your brow* is the manifestation of your effort to subject the fallen elements of your body to your divine spirit.

LINE UPON LINE SUMMARY

On Your Marks

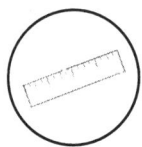 Receive God's image. Remember, your body is *the measure of your creation*—the physical manifestation of your potential to become like God.

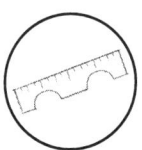 Yoke yourself to Christ when you exercise. Remember, *His yoke will enable* the measure of your creation to be filled with a fulness of joy.

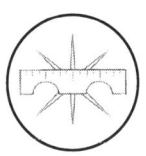 Invite the Spirit to be with you when you exercise. Remember, *His power will quicken* the measure of your creation so you can experience a fulness of joy.

LINE UPON LINE SUMMARY

Get Set

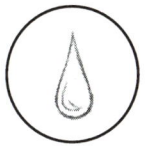 Sweat in the wilderness of regular exercise. The *sweat of your brow* is the manifestation of your effort to subject the fallen elements of your body to your divine spirit.

CHAPTER 5

Defend against the Adversary's Fiery Darts

The crowd of middle school students and their parents gasped in disbelief at what they had just witnessed. In the moments prior to this spectacle, the middle school principal had listed the various accomplishments that the winner of this award had achieved during the last year of school. When my name was announced, I felt a surge of pride fill my whole being. I left my seat next to my mother and walked nonchalantly toward the auditorium stage like a prizefighter to the ring, giving high fives to my friends while I soaked in the crowd's applause. All that was between me and my trophy was the stage steps. A prideful thought penetrated my expanding head. *Take them triumphantly, two at a time.* This temptation seemed the right thing to do, considering the occasion. So I increased my speed and bounded upward, skipping the first step and misjudging the second. My momentum threw me forward. I reached out to brace myself and crashed hard onto the stage floor. For what seemed like minutes, though only mere seconds, I lay facedown on the stage as my peers and their parents held their breath.

I couldn't believe what had just happened. I began to feel a burning sensation in my right shin; however, it was a mere annoyance when compared to the embarrassment that was crushing my ego. My middle school life was over. That misstep had just inscribed my legacy in the middle school's hall of shame forever. I cautiously pressed my throbbing hands down into the stage and quickly realized I had put myself in a very familiar position. My wise father found great success in making pushups a form of discipline in our home. Our extended family rumored that they could easily critique which one of us boys had the more rebellious-filled summer based upon our muscular physique.

So, true to form and in a desperate attempt to recover a bit of my glory, I decided to do a few pushups. It worked! With each pushup, the crowd began to giggle. After a few more, their giggles turned into outright laughs. Once I felt that their laughter was greater than my embarrassment, I got up off the floor and accepted my trophy—a large piece of humble pie that had inscribed on it the words, "Eighth Grade Athlete of the Year." I quickly and carefully exited the stage, found my mother, and whispered into her ear, "Can we go home now?" She smiled, patted my knee, and wisely said, "Let's stay and support the rest of your classmates."

DEFEND

Think back to Christ's wilderness experience. After His forty days and forty nights communing with and learning from the Father about how to more completely subject His mortal body to His divine spirit, Satan thrice came to tempt Him to use His newly gained power to exercise unrighteous dominion over the elements (see Matthew 4:3–11). Satan will do the same as you exercise to increase your physical capacity to fill the measure of your creation with joy. In order to defend against his fiery darts of temptation (the darts that led to my eighth grade fall), we must first understand why he desires our destruction.

> And I, the Lord God, spake unto Moses, saying: That Satan, whom thou hast commanded in the name of mine Only Begotten, is the same which was from the beginning, and he came before me, saying—Behold, here am I, send me, I will be thy son, and I will redeem *all mankind*, that *one soul shall not be lost*, and surely I will do it; wherefore *give me* thine honor. . . .
>
> Wherefore, because that Satan rebelled against me, and *sought to destroy the agency of man*, which I, the Lord God, had given him, and

Defend against the Adversary's Fiery Darts

also, that I should *give unto him mine own power; by the power of mine Only Begotten*, I caused that he should be cast down;

And he became Satan, yea, even the devil, the father of all *lies*, to deceive and to blind men, and to lead them captive at his will, even as many as would not hearken unto my voice. (Moses 4:1, 3–4; emphasis added)

These verses reveal that Satan's premortal plan was to destroy the agency of man so he could obtain the power of God's Only Begotten. His personal plan of pride promised that not one soul would be lost. However, herein lies the foundational lie of his premortal plan. If our agency were destroyed, there would have been no purpose for our creation. We would be unable to choose between good and evil, thus eliminating our susceptibility to sin and our ability to become like our Father (see 2 Nephi 2:11–13). If we could not sin, there would be no need for God's Only Begotten to sacrifice His body and blood in our behalf. Satan's premortal plan was *all about him!* There was no thought or concern for us. Satan wanted one thing: He wanted the power that came with being the Only Begotten Son of God—the power of an immortal, with an exalted physical body like our Father in Heaven's. With this power, he could fulfill the desire of his heart to "ascend into heaven," to "exalt [his] throne above the stars of God," to "ascend above the heights of the clouds," and to "be like the most High" (Isaiah 14:12–14).

Satan's personal plan of pride would exalt only one. In contrast, the Father's plan required the sacrifice of one who would provide the opportunity for all to be exalted. The choice was clear; our Father chose the first and the *most fit* of His spirit children to be His Only Begotten, our Savior, Jesus Christ, who from the beginning sought only the will of our Father. "But, behold, my Beloved Son, which was my Beloved and Chosen from the beginning, said unto me—Father, thy will be done, and the glory be thine forever" (Moses 4:2).

With God's choice confirmed, Satan's premortal plan of pride was rejected. In his wrath, a war commenced, and Satan continued to propagandize his plan to deceive God's children. The Apostle John wrote the following about this war:

> And there was war in heaven: Michael and his angels fought against the dragon; and the dragon fought and his angels,
>
> And prevailed not; neither was their place found any more in heaven.
>
> And the great dragon was cast out, that old serpent, called the Devil, and Satan, which deceiveth the whole world: he was cast out into the earth, and his angels were cast out with him. (Revelation 12:7–9)

Satan was cast out *without* the one thing he desired most—a physical body. He and his minions were cast down to earth, the very place that was prepared for God's children to experience mortality. Satan's choice to rebel against God made him eternally *unfit* for the blessing of God's Kingdom. Elder David A. Bednar of the Quorum of the Twelve Apostles describes Satan's unfit state in this way:

> Satan does not have a body, and his eternal progress has been halted. Just as water flowing in a riverbed is stopped by a dam, so the adversary's eternal progress is thwarted because he does not have a physical body. Because of his rebellion, Lucifer has denied himself all of the mortal blessings and experiences *made possible through a tabernacle of flesh and bones*. He cannot learn the lessons that only an embodied spirit can learn. He cannot marry or enjoy the blessings of procreation and family life. He cannot abide the reality of a literal and universal resurrection of all mankind. One of the potent scriptural meanings of the word *damned* [italics in original] is illustrated in his inability to continue developing and becoming like our Heavenly Father.[1]

Satan's mandated misery as a disembodied spirit led the Apostle John to warn us, saying, "*Woe* to the inhabiters of the earth and of the sea! for the devil is come down unto you, *having great wrath*, because he knoweth that he hath but a short time" (Revelation 12:12; emphasis added).

Satan has a short time to do what? The Apostle John reveals Satan's desires: "And [Satan] opened his mouth . . . to blaspheme *his name*, and his *tabernacle*" (Revelation 13:6; emphasis added). Satan's purpose on this earth is to blaspheme and destroy, if possible, that which he can never have, the title (*name*) and body (*tabernacle*) of God's Only Begotten Son. Because you and I have taken upon us the name of Christ and have a body of flesh and bones that is "in similitude" of the Only Begotten,

Defend against the Adversary's Fiery Darts

Satan desires to have us (see 3 Nephi 18:18). To get us, he tempts us to blaspheme the name of Christ and to destroy the very bodies God has given us! Satan does this by exercising dominion over the elements of our bodies in a manner that is contrary to the purpose of their creation—to live in similitude of Him.

GET SET

All of the fiery darts that Satan hurls our way are to ignite the carnal kerosene of our fallen natures. There are three specific fiery darts that the adversary is using to tempt us to blaspheme our bodies (see Revelation 13:6) with great success in the latter days. They are the fiery darts of physical *lust, latency,* and *limits.*

The most propagandized of the three is the fiery dart of physical *lust.* Satan knows that our bodies have been created to experience opposition, such as pleasure and pain, health and sickness, and sorrow and joy so that we can become like God (see Genesis 3:22). Physical lust is the natural man's desire to swap our birthright of immortal and eternal happiness for a meager bowl of mortality's pulses of pleasure (see Genesis 25:29–34). With this fiery dart, Satan tempts us to dine with him and eat the pottage when we "*misuse* [our] physical tabernacles by violating the law of chastity, by using drugs and addictive substances, by disfiguring or defacing [ourselves], or by worshipping the false idol of body image, whether [our] own or that of others."[2] Lust is the fiery dart that lures us to *misuse* our physical bodies and, by doing so, eventually *refuse* our birthright—eternal life (see D&C 88:28–32).

Physical *latency* is one of Satan's more pernicious darts, an often imperceptible dart that starts a slow-burning fire that can "pacify, and lull [us] away into carnal security" (2 Nephi 28:21), enticing us to "eat, drink, and be merry . . . for tomorrow we die" (2 Nephi 28:8). Satan knows that our bodies constitute our second estate (see Abraham 3:26)—the state that enables us to act rather than to be acted upon. Satan seeks to foreclose our second estate by tempting us "to *disconnect* gradually and *physically* from things as they really are. In essence, he encourages us to think and act as if we were in our premortal, *unembodied* state."[3] One of the most powerful ways that the adversary does this is by tempting us to take up our primary residence in the cloud of virtual technology. This cloud is not evil in and of itself; however, when we spend hours each day streaming, updating, hashtagging, tweeting, and acting in a virtual form, we run the risk of disconnecting from our bodies (the measure of our creation), thus taking up a mental and emotional residence in a "great and spacious [virtual] building . . . high above the earth" (see 1 Nephi 8:26).

Now consider how successful Satan has been in tempting the children of God to take up residence in his condos of virtual captivity. According to the Centers for Disease Control and Prevention, roughly 80 percent of American adults do not exercise regularly, and 25 percent are not active at all.[4] This statistic is derived from the fact that we, on average, expose ourselves to virtual screens—TVs, computers, mobile devices—for more than eight hours on any given day! Satan's plan is an on demand, high definition, and instant messaging temptation to "set at naught" our bodies by *not using* them (see 1 Nephi 19:7). The adversary knows that when we are disconnected from the virtue of our mortal reality, the dust of physical latency will settle upon us (see Isaiah 52:2) and gradually decrease our physical desire and capacity to act upon the elements of our body. A decrease in our physical desire increases his power to act upon us.

Physical *limits* are the most logical of Satan's fiery darts. This dart fuels the mindset that it is impossible, or at least too difficult, to exercise dominion over the elements of our bodies. Laman and Lemuel were often burned by this fiery dart. When commanded of the Lord to return to Jerusalem to obtain the plates, they murmured, saying it was a "hard thing" that God required of them (1 Nephi 3:5). When Nephi's bow broke and their bows had lost their spring, making it "difficult" to obtain food, they complained against the Lord (see 1 Nephi 16:21–22). When Nephi was commanded of the Lord to build a ship, Laman and Lemuel belittled their brother, bearing false witness of his physical capacity by saying that "our brother is a fool, for he thinketh that he can build a ship; yea, and he also thinketh that he can cross these great waters" (1 Nephi 17:17).

Defend against the Adversary's Fiery Darts

Laman and Lemuel's chronic acceptance of Satan's lie of physical limits filled the measure of their creation with more murmuring than it did joy. The same can happen to us. Limiting mind-sets, such as "I was made this way" and "I don't have time to exercise," are some of the fiery darts that the adversary uses to keep us from exercising dominion over our bodies.

Satan sends his fiery darts of physical lust, latency, and limitations to derail and cause our fitness efforts to fail. In the following scriptures, the Lord has lovingly taught us how to defend against these darts and keep them from igniting our carnal natures:

- Behold, verily, verily, I say unto you, ye must *watch and pray* always lest ye enter into temptation; for Satan desireth to have you, that he may sift you as wheat. (3 Nephi 18:18; emphasis added)
- *Watch and pray*, that ye enter not into temptation: the spirit indeed *is* [italics in original] willing, but the flesh *is* [italics in original] weak. (Matthew 26:41; emphasis added)
- But that ye would humble yourselves before the Lord, and call on his holy name, and *watch and pray* continually, that ye may not be tempted above that which ye can bear, and thus be led by the Holy Spirit, becoming humble, meek, submissive, patient, full of love and all long-suffering. (Alma 13:28; emphasis added)

Remember, Satan's plan is to tempt you to blaspheme the name of Christ and the body God has given you, to act in a manner that will fill the measure of your creation with misery. Like Captain Moroni, you can protect yourself by building a mental "tower"—a "[place] of security" (Alma 50:4–5) that will enable you to safely *watch* for the fiery darts that the adversary will hurl to derail your efforts to get physically *fit for good*.

You can begin to build your mental "place of security" by writing your answers to the two simple questions below.

1. Why do I *really* want to get fit?

_____
_____
_____
_____
_____
_____
_____

2. What is *really* keeping me from getting fit?

_____
_____
_____
_____
_____
_____
_____

Now take a good look at your answers. Look for ways that the adversary might use them to light the carnal kerosene that fuels your natural man. For example, if you really want to get fit to feel good, that is a great place to start. However, watch out! The adversary will use his fiery dart of physical lust to tempt you to move your motive from getting fit to feel good physically to getting fit to feel good about yourself because you look good. This dart can burn a scarring connection between your self-worth and your physical appearance.

Look at what is keeping you from getting fit. Does a perceived lack of time, lack of energy, or lack of desire provide the perfect kindling for the adversary's immobilizing darts of physical latency and limitations? Watch out for Satan's darts that can be used to damn your fitness efforts.

Defend against the Adversary's Fiery Darts

Then, as you're watching out for Satan's darts, remember to pray! Call upon the Lord for the wisdom to discern and the strength to defend against these fiery darts that will derail your efforts to get *fit for good*. Ask for guidance to not look beyond the mark that is the measure of your creation. Seek to be yoked to Christ, and invite the Spirit to be with you as you exercise. By doing this, you will prepare yourself to build your body upon the rock of your Redeemer, "that when the devil shall send forth his mighty winds, yea, his shafts in the whirlwind, yea, when all his hail and his mighty storm shall beat upon you, it shall have no power over you to drag you down to the gulf of misery and endless wo, because of the rock upon which ye are built, which is a sure foundation, a foundation whereon if men build they cannot fall" (Helaman 5:12).

Defend against the adversary's fiery darts. *Watch and pray* for protection against the darts of physical lust, latency, and limits that will fill the measure of your creation with misery.

LINE UPON LINE SUMMARY

On Your Mark

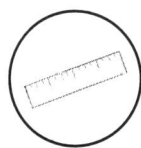

Receive God's image. Remember, your body is *the measure of your creation*—the physical manifestation of your potential to become like God.

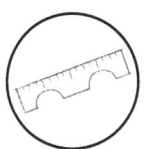

Yoke yourself to Christ when you exercise. Remember, *His yoke will enable* the measure of your creation to be filled with a fulness of joy.

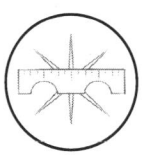

Invite the Spirit to be with you when you exercise. Remember, *His power will quicken* the measure of your creation so you can experience a fulness of joy.

Defend against the Adversary's Fiery Darts

LINE UPON LINE SUMMARY

Get Set

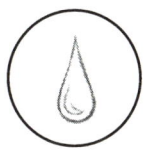
Sweat in the wilderness of regular exercise. The *sweat of your brow* is the manifestation of your effort to subject the fallen elements of your body to your divine spirit.

Defend against the adversary's fiery darts. *Watch and pray* for protection against the darts of physical lust, latency, and limits that will fill the measure of your creation with misery.

CHAPTER 6

Experiment upon the Word of God

I was grateful for the time I had to study. In a few days, I would be taking my physical therapy boards. I sat at the far end of the YMCA gymnastics gym, occasionally looking up to watch my daughter Tay, now six years old, participate in her gymnastics class. Her instructor suggested that she transition to the more advanced group. Tay quickly scurried over to where I was sitting and asked my permission. I answered in the affirmative. With an excited bounce in her step, she ran back to her instructor to tell her the good news.

At this point, my studies didn't seem as important as keeping a close eye on my little girl. I watched as she experienced the beam, the vault, and the floor for the first time. She beamed from ear to ear after completing very basic maneuvers on each apparatus. Her instructor then escorted the group to the uneven bars just a few feet from where I was sitting. The students lined up as one of the older, taller, and more experienced gymnasts demonstrated what the students would be doing. The gymnast swung herself around the low bar and, with the aid of the instructor, propped herself up on it. She then leaped forward through the air and grabbed the high bar, swinging back and forth until she came to a graceful stop.

My eyes instantly grew two sizes. *There is no way Tay can make that jump,* I thought to myself. *She's way too little.* My daughter was blessed with her mother's grace—and my short stature. I looked her way; she was nervously fidgeting and rubbing her hands together. We both watched as student after student attempted the feat. Very few were successful. Most were caught by the instructor and her aide. The line quickly disappeared in front of my anxious little girl. She glanced over at me. I flashed her a less-than-confident smile. Instantly, she ran toward me. I opened my arms, expecting her to break down in tears. However, she stopped in front of me, held my outstretched hand, and asked, "Do you think I can do it, Dad?" I was so caught off guard that I blurted out, "I know you can do it." She gave me a quick hug and returned to her place in line. *What have I just done?* I thought to myself. *I just lied to my daughter!* She looked over at me, took a deep breath, and gave me a thumbs-up.

Her turn finally came. The aide helped hoist her up onto the low bar. *Please catch her,* I thought to myself. She carefully crouched down and at the instructor's command launched herself off the low bar. I watched my little girl launch forward like a flying squirrel through the air, right before my eyes. She caught hold of the high bar with ease. She dangled from the high bar, her face beaming with confidence, as she waited for her instructor to help her down. She ran back to the end of the line and gave me another thumbs-up. I closed my dropped jaw and gave her one back.

EXPERIMENT

Why was my little squirrel of a girl able to complete such an amazing feat? It was because she chose to exercise *faith* in the words of her father. In the Prophet Joseph Smith's *Lectures on Faith,* we learn the following truth:

> If men were duly to consider themselves, and turn their thoughts and reflections to the operations of their own minds, they would readily discover that it is faith, and *faith only*, which is the *moving cause of all action, in them; that without it, both mind and body would be in a state of inactivity*, and all their exertions would cease, both physical and mental.

Experiment upon the Word of God

Were this class to go back and reflect upon the history of their lives, from the period of their first recollection, and ask themselves, *what principle excited them to action, or what gave them energy and activity.* . . . What would be the answer? . . . Turn your thoughts on your own minds, and *see if faith is not the moving cause of all action* in yourselves.[1]

Faith is the moving cause of all action in men! Let me say that again. *Faith is the moving cause of all action in men!* Therefore, whenever you are physically active—or in other words, moving—you are exercising faith. Every year, millions of people exercise sufficient faith to claim the promise of increased physical fitness by the sweat of regular physical exercise. You can see this every Saturday morning on the infomercials that project the thousands of before-and-after videos, pictures, and testimonials of those whose "sweat-based" faith physically transformed, or "converted," their bodies. However, here lies the problem: Their physical fitness conversions normally do not last. The percentage that maintain their physical conversions for more than a year is less than 20 percent, with nearly 70 percent regaining more weight within five years of their initial transformation.[2] Why? It's because a lasting physical fitness "conversion" only comes when the "sweat" of our brow beads as we exercise faith in the word of God, not in a man-made fitness program, product, or process.

There are three things that are necessary for us to exercise faith in the word of God "unto life and salvation":

First the idea that [God] actually exists.

Secondly, a *correct* idea of [God's] character, perfections and attributes.

Thirdly, an actual knowledge that the course of life which [one] is pursuing is according to his will. For without an acquaintance with these three important facts, the faith of every rational being must be imperfect and unproductive; but with this understanding, it can become perfect and fruitful.[3]

These three principles relate to the eternal marks you stepped to in part one. Those marks make it possible for you to exercise faith in the word of God as you exercise. When you *first* receive God's image, you will accept the idea that God physically exists. *Secondly*, when you choose to exercise yoked to Christ, you will learn of Him (see Alma 38:9) and gain a correct idea of God's character, perfections, and attributes. *Thirdly*, when you invite the Spirit to be a part or your exercise efforts, His companionship will witness that the course of life you are pursuing is in accordance with God's will. These three eternal marks are the foundation that will enable you to "exercise" faith in the word of God to increase your physical capacity to fill the measure of your creation with joy.

Let's return one last time to Christ's wilderness experience to better understand the relationship between the word of God and our physical bodies. Elder James E. Talmage of the Quorum of the Twelve wrote the following words:

> When [Christ] was hungry and physically weak, the tempter came with the insidious suggestion that He use His extraordinary powers to provide food. Satan had chosen the most propitious time for his evil purpose. What will mortals not do, to what lengths have men not gone, to assuage the pangs of hunger? Esau bartered his birthright for a meal. Men have fought like brutes for food. Women have slain and eaten their own babes rather than endure the gnawing pangs of starvation. All this Satan knew when he came to the Christ in the hour of extreme physical need, and said unto Him: "If thou be the Son of God, command that these stones be made bread."[4]

Satan's temptation was twofold: one, to tempt Christ to *prove* that he had dominion over the elements, and two, to tempt Him to *succumb* to the elements of His hungered and weakened body. Satan tempted the Savior to give up all He had gained in His wilderness experience by exercising *unrighteous* dominion over the elements of His body.

In Christ's response to Satan's temptations, we discover the relationship between our bodies and the word of God. Christ responded by reciting a scripture found in Deuteronomy chapter 8. In this particular verse, the Lord revealed to Moses why He had led the children of Israel throughout the wilderness for forty years. The Lord explained that it was to "humble" and "prove" them, that they might "know that man doth not *live by* bread only, but by *every word* that proceedeth out of the mouth of the Lord doth man *live*." (Deuteronomy 8:2–3; emphasis added). Christ, in His response to Satan's flesh-focused temptation, boldly declared and revealed to each of us that the physical elements of our bodies are not sustained by the partaking of bread (*physical nourishment*) alone, but that our bodies are sustained moment to moment by the very word of God (see Mosiah 2:21).

The elements of our bodies function because of His word. Consider your diaphragm and your heart. From your first breath to this very moment, they have been contracting to oxygenate and pump blood through nearly sixty thousand miles of vessels in your body, a distance equivalent to more than two trips around the world. These vessels deliver oxygen, energy, and nutrients to each of the estimated seventy trillion cells in your body so they might complete their very specialized work that God commands them to perform. At the same time, billions of brain cells are firing impulses to every part of your body as you read and comprehend these words, while roaming immune cells throughout your body are on constant guard, looking for and neutralizing the countless pathogens that seek to cause you harm. These amazing processes occur with *no conscious effort* of your own. What directs them to function in such a miraculous manner? The very word of God! You and I are breathing, walking, seeing, and speaking beings that *live by* and *because of* the word of God.

GET SET

Remember the story about my little girl? It was her choice to *live by* her father's words that enabled her to master the elements of her little body and successfully leap toward and grasp onto the high bar. You can do the same to master the elements of your physical body. This is done through scripture mastery. I'm not talking about the diligent study and memorization of scripture, though such mastery is important. I am talking about *mastering* ourselves through scripture. This is done when we choose to "awake and arouse [our] faculties" to *experiment* upon the words of our Father in Heaven (Alma 32:27).

I have participated in several clinical research experiments that have been presented at various physical therapy conferences and published in various journals. In these experiments, I have sought to discover ways to help physical therapists and their patients learn how to better "exercise dominion" over the elements of their physical bodies in order to decrease pain and improve body function. Professionals establish the value and validity of any experiment when other researchers know they can re-create the experiment over and over again with the same outcome—when the outcome of the experiment is known, but not yet seen (see Hebrews 11:1). This can only happen if those who are performing the experiment follow the same pattern as exemplified by the original author.

Just like researchers can try the same experiment to get the same results, there is a divine pattern found in the word of God that you can experiment upon to exercise righteous dominion over the elements of your body. It is the pattern established by the "author and finisher of our faith" (Hebrews 12:2) as He exercised dominion over the elements of the universe to frame the world that you and I live upon by the power of His Word (see Hebrews 11:3). In part three of this book, you will be invited to "awake and arouse your faculties" to "experiment" upon His word (Alma 32:27) by following the Lord's pattern of creation as found in the holy scriptures. This divine pattern will teach you *how* to exercise dominion over the elements of your body and increase your physical capacity to fill the measure of your creation with joy.

 Experiment upon the word of God. By *exercising faith in the word of God*, you can increase your physical capacity to fill the measure of your creation with a fulness of joy.

LINE UPON LINE SUMMARY

On Your Mark

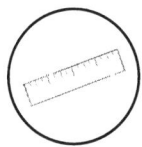
Receive God's image. Remember, your body is *the measure of your creation*—the physical manifestation of your potential to become like God.

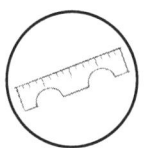
Yoke yourself to Christ when you exercise. Remember, *His yoke will enable* the measure of your creation to be filled with a fulness of joy.

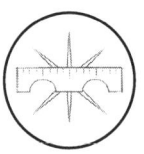
Invite the Spirit to be with you when you exercise. Remember, *His power will quicken* the measure of your creation so you can experience a fulness of joy.

LINE UPON LINE SUMMARY

Get Set

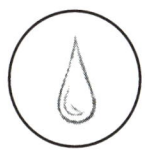

Sweat in the wilderness of regular exercise. The *sweat of your brow* is the manifestation of your effort to subject the fallen elements of your body to your divine spirit.

Defend against the adversary's fiery darts. *Watch and pray* for protection against the darts of physical lust, latency, and limits that will fill the measure of your creation with misery.

Experiment upon the word of God. By *exercising faith in the word of God*, you can increase your physical capacity to fill the measure of your creation with a fulness of joy.

PART THREE

Go!

The race has been marked. You are set. Now is the time to go! When the starter gave the command to go, the runners acted upon the elements of their body in various ways. Some started by leading with their left leg, others with their right. Some grimaced and grunted as others kept stoic and silent. Each individual's pattern of movement propelled them forward. My personal pattern was initially very effective, as evident by my quick burst to the front of the pack. However, in time, it failed me. Part three of *Fit for Good* will help you experiment upon the word of God as patterned in the Creation. That divine pattern will form, divide, beautify, and multiply your physical fitness. That divine pattern will enable you to become physically *fit for good*.

CHAPTER 7
Create a Fitness Focus

I had dreamt about this exact moment for years. I had laid the foundation for this moment over hours of practice. I was about to see this amazing athlete fill the measure of his creation, and a portion of mine, in a single feat of greatness. His physical *form* was perfect inside his bright blue uniform. My body tensed with excitement as I watched this athlete *divide* the soccer ball from the feet of the opposing team's best player. I couldn't hold it in any longer. My voice broke through the cheers of the crowd as I yelled, "Go! Go! Go to the goal!" Following my obnoxious cue, he began to dribble toward the soccer goal. It was a thing of *beauty* watching him exercise such skilful dominion over the elements of his body. All that separated him from the goal was twenty yards of green grass.

My pulse matched his quickening pace as I contemplated the consequences that would come from this critical moment. Greatness would be witnessed, a hero would be born, and the future of athletic success would be secured if only . . . my four-year-old son could score his first soccer goal.

My heart suddenly stopped. The player he had taken the ball away from was now in hot pursuit. Her long blonde pigtails trailed behind her focused face that witnessed of her determination to reclaim that which she had lost. My excitement quickly turned into concern as my eyes darted back and forth between my son and this driven little girl. She was gaining on him!

Like most four-year-olds, my son came to a standstill just a few yards in front of the goal to "power up" his kick. It was too late. The pigtails in hot pursuit had arrived. My dream seemed doomed; however, a sliver of hope came by way of this little girl's momentum. Unable to control it, she clipped my son's back leg and sent her petite frame careening toward the ground in a conglomerate of flaying arms, legs, and pigtails. Had the windows of heaven opened? My son now had an uncontested shot at the goal. I tried to yell to shoot; however, like the lions in the den with Daniel, the Lord mercifully shut my mouth so that I might witness the moment when my son would fulfil the measure of his creation. He looked at the ball, the goal, and then at the little pigtailed girl who was now curled up on the ground in a ball of tears.

He gave up the goal and went to the girl. He gently helped her to her feet, patted her on the shoulder, and said a few kind words. She wiped her tears as a sweet smile surfaced on her face and then on my son's. The smiles began to *multiply* on the faces of all those who had witnessed this simple yet sacred event. The on-field coaches then encouraged them to play on.

CREATE

In that moment, my son provided all who were watching a perfect example of *how* we can physically exercise to fill the measure of our creation with a fulness of joy. He had exercised dominion over the elements of his body according to the Lord's divine pattern of creation—the pattern of *forming, dividing, beautifying,* and *multiplying* that will enable you to become physically *fit for good*.

In the first phase of the Creation, the Lord *formed* the earth. "And the Lord said: Let us go down. And they went down at the beginning, and they, that is the Gods, organized and *formed* the heavens and the earth" (Abraham 4:1; emphasis added).

Create a Fitness Focus

In the second phase, God *divided* the earth. "And I, God, said: Let there be light; and there was light. And I, God, saw the light; and that light was good. And I, God, *divided* the light form the darkness. . . . And again, I, God, said: Let there be a firmament in the midst of the water, and it was so, even as I spake; and I said: Let it *divide* the waters from the waters; and it was done" (Moses 2:3–4, 6; emphasis added).

In the third phase, God *beautified* the earth. "And the earth brought forth grass, every herb yielding seed after his kind, and the tree yielding fruit, whose seed should be in itself, after his kind; and I, God, saw that all things which I had made were *good*" (Moses 2:12; emphasis added).

All three of the previous phases were completed *for* the final phase of Creation, the phase in which God invited His children to *multiply* upon the earth. "And I, God, created man . . . And I, God, blessed them, and said unto them: Be fruitful, and *multiply*, and replenish the earth, and subdue it, and have dominion over . . . every living thing that moveth upon the earth" (Moses 2:27–28; emphasis added).

We find within the final phase of the Creation the fulness of God's purpose. The understanding of this purpose, the reason why our Father does all that He does, is the anchor that will enable you to experiment upon His pattern of creation and become physically *fit for good*.

Over the last thousand years or so, mankind, both believers and non-believers, have discussed and debated *how* the earth was created. The answer to this question will forever be fruitless until we ask the question *why*—to understand the *purpose* for which it was created. The same holds true in your efforts to exercise dominion over the elements of your body. If you spend your time and resources focusing on *how* to become physically fit while never truly understanding *why* you want to get fit, you run the risk of building your body on a sandy foundation—a foundation that will shift, settle, and eventually wash away under the downpours of mortality (see 3 Nephi 14:26–27).

You can discover what your purpose is by practicing what can be called *whyse discernment*. Whyse discernment is the act of asking the question "*why*" again and again until you become "*wise*" to the fundamental reason why you are doing something.

I was first introduced to whyse discernment, and invited to practice it, by my wife when she asked me why I had run in the boot race. For the sake of demonstration, let me show how the practice of whyse discernment could have helped me discover the fundamental purpose of my promenade down "Whiskey Row."

My wife: *Why* did you run the race?

Me: Because I wanted to see if I could win it.

My wife: *Why* did you want to win it?

Me: Because I wanted my family and friends to see me win.

My wife: *Why* did you want them to see you win?

Me: Because I wanted to impress them.

My wife: *Why* did you want to impress them?

Me: Because I wanted them to compliment me.

My wife: *Why* did you want them to compliment you?

Me: Because when people compliment me, I feel accepted.

My wife: *Why* do you want to feel accepted?

Me: Because when I feel accepted, *I'm happy*.

With six *whyse* questions, I uncovered the fundamental purpose of why I ran the race—to be happy! In the previous chapter, you began to practice whyse discernment when you answered the question, "Why do I want to get fit?" I am sure that your answer was one or two whyse questions away (rather than six away) from this fundamental purpose. In fact, I'm confident your answer had something to do with feeling good—the physical description of happiness.

Remember, "Happiness is *the purpose* and design of our existence 'Men are that they might have joy.'"[1] President Dieter F. Uchtdorf of the First Presidency declared that "our *birthright*—and the *purpose* of our great voyage on this earth—is *to seek and experience eternal happiness*."[2] This is why the Lord created the earth, so that we might have a place to

Create a Fitness Focus

learn how to fill the measures of our creation with a fulness of joy (see Abraham 3:24). It is the same reason why you want to get physically fit—to be happy and have joy.

Consider this critical truth: the selfless good Samaritan and the selfish criminal do what they do for the same purpose—to experience joy. However, here is the key difference: the measure of joy that will be meted from their works will be very different. The criminal will have a measure of "joy in [his] works for a season, [but] by and by the end cometh" (3 Nephi 27:11) and the measure of his creation will be found wanting for more (see Isaiah 29:8). The good Samaritan will not be found wanting because he chose to invest his efforts not in robbing this certain man's "earthly treasures" (Matthew 6:19), but in the service of him. His investment was to "lay up treasures in heaven" (Matthew 6:20) where the return will undoubtedly be a fulness of joy in this life and the life to come.

The same holds true for our exercise efforts. We are all trying to get physically fit to fill the measure of our creation with joy. However, the measure of joy that will be meted unto us will ultimately be determined by what motivates our fitness behaviors.

GO!

Each phase of the Creation metes a specific measure of joy and bestows a specific blessing that will increase your physical capacity to fill the measure of your creation with joy. We will discuss the blessings of each phase in the following chapters. However, it is critical to first understand the measure of joy each phase will mete in order to defend against the adversary who, with his fiery darts, will try to undermine and frustrate your efforts to get physically *fit for good*. This understanding can come from the Motivational Matrix on the next page.

Fit for Good

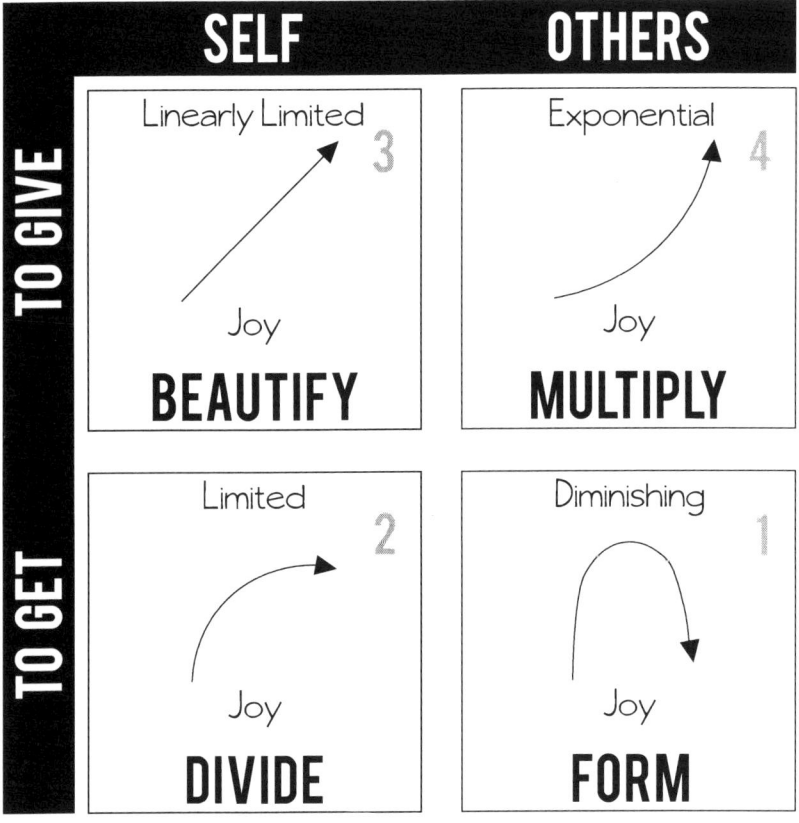

As you can see, the measure of joy we can receive from our fitness efforts is dependent upon what we are getting fit for. For example, if your exercise efforts are focused on getting fit to primarily improve your physical features, then you are getting fit for the joy found in the first phase of the Creation, the forming phase. The joy we often seek in this phase is primarily the praise or acceptance we *get* from *another person* because of our more physically fit form. The measure of joy meted in this phase will always fade, like how the summer in which you found joy in that slimming swimsuit fades into fall.

We will discuss in greater detail the diminishing, limited, linearly limited, and exponential measures of joy we gain from each quadrant of the matrix in the following chapters. In order to overcome fitness failure, your exercise efforts must be focused on claiming not the joy, but the hidden

Create a Fitness Focus

blessing found in each of the first three phases. These specific blessings will increase your physical capacity to participate in and thus experience the fulness of joy found only in the fourth. The adversary will use his fiery darts to keep you from receiving the exponential joy of the fourth by tempting you to focus your exercise efforts on filling the measure of your creation with the unfulfilling joy rather than on obtaining the specific blessings of the first three phases. The key to becoming physically *fit for good*, is to claim the blessings of the first three phases to increase your physical capacity to participate in the fourth phase, to *give* of yourself to *others* in order to fill the measure of your creation with a fulness of joy (see Matthew 16:25). The fourth quadrant is the quadrant where our Father in Heaven functions. He does all that He does to *give* "immortality and eternal life" to His children (Moses 1:39).

This divine declaration is the *focus* of all His works. It is why He *moves* upon the elements of the universe to give us the opportunity to become like Him—to have an immortal body that has the capacity to receive a fulness of joy. Before you begin to experiment upon the Lord's pattern of creation, you will need to create a personal *fitness focus* statement that will help you stay focused on claiming the specific blessings of the first three phases so that you can fully participate in the final phase, the phase that will fill the measure of your creation with a fulness of joy and enable you to become *fit for good*.

Start first by remembering the eternal marks we discussed in part one. You have been physically measured, yoked, and quickened for a purpose. Focus your fitness efforts by counseling with your Father (Alma 37:37) and asking Him this question: *What would Thou have me be physically fit for?* Read, pray, and ponder over this question. As thoughts come to your mind, record them below.

_____

_____

_____

_____

Fit for Good

_____
_____
_____
_____
_____
_____
_____
_____

Look at the revelation you received above and work to whittle it into a personal, short, and simple fitness focus statement. If you are struggling with this, follow the Lord's example of declaring the focus of His "work and glory" (Moses 1:39) by filling in the blank below.

For behold, I will get and stay physically fit _____ .

Here are a few examples:

Physically fit for good.
Physically fit for the fruition of the Lord's work.
Physically fit to feel good so I can do good.
Physically fit to be a light for others.
Physically fit for the kingdom.
Physically fit to follow Him.
Physically fit to serve.
Physically moving to make a difference.
Physically buff enough to bear another's burden.

When ready, please record your fitness focus statement on the following lines.

Create a Fitness Focus

_____
_____
_____
_____
_____
_____

What you have written above will likely be focused on the fourth quadrant, getting fit to *give* to *others,* the only quadrant with the exponential joy that can motivate you to get and stay physically *fit for good*.

For example, consider the man who sleeps warm in bed but is awoken by the alarm he set for 6:00 a.m. to exercise. His body balks at the idea of leaving the comfort of his bed to exercise; however, his desire to exercise is motivated by the power of God's word. He recites his fitness focus statement: *I sweat to serve.* He glances over at the sleeping beauty lying next to him and thinks of the four children that they have together. Motivated by his fitness focus, he moves upon the carnally content and bed-bound elements of his body and heads out the door to fill the measure of his creation with the joy of *sweating to serve.* Consider the woman who stands in front of the rack of exercise clothes at the store. She peruses through various options, many which would jeopardize her convictions of modesty. She recalls her fitness focus: *I will get physically fit for the fruition of the Lord's work.* She chooses not to stray from it and selects an outfit that won't "check her religion at the door" of the gym, but instead witnesses her desire to get *fit for the fruition of the Lord's work.*[3]

With your fitness focus established, you are now ready to practice the eternal principle that will enable you to claim the specific blessings associated with each phase of the Creation. It is "what we learn in the temple—the *return-and-report* principle."[4] This principle is the act of returning and reporting to someone else our efforts to fulfill the errands given to us from the Lord. For example, when we return and report our home or visiting teaching to the Elders Quorum or Relief Society president, we are following the return-and-report principle. It is a principle that keeps us connected to the Lord.

We find the power of this principle in the words of President Thomas S. Monson. He taught that "when performance is *measured* and *reported*, the rate of improvement accelerates."[5] This combination of measuring and reporting on your efforts to exercise according to your fitness focus will enable you to become *fit for good*.

Many people try to measure their fitness progress with each glance in a mirror, step on a scale, measure of the waist, or pinch of skin. However, they often forfeit any improvements that they see through these measures because they fail to focus and report on their reasons for getting fit.

A Fitness Focus Sphere will help you to measure your efforts to get physically fit and record your efforts in each phase of the Creation over a four-week cycle. Here is a copy, and you can download it at physicallyfitforgood.com. You will learn how to use it in detail as we work our way through each chapter.

Create a Fitness Focus

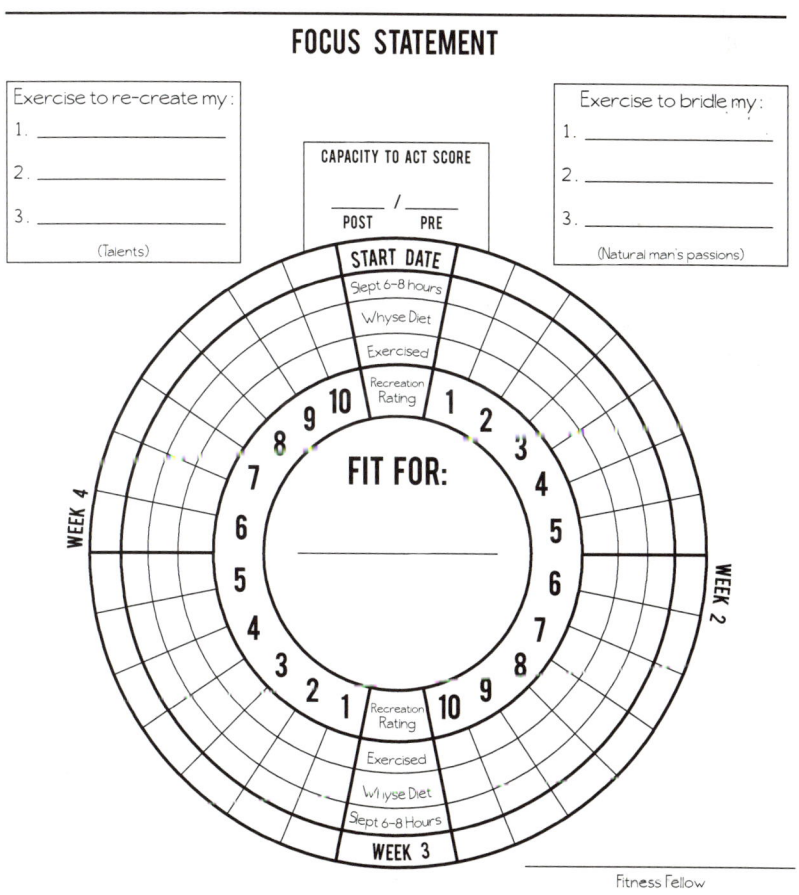

Fit for Good

The Fitness Focus Sphere will help keep you focused on your purpose. However, you will need a *fitness fellow* to help you report on your fitness efforts. Choose someone that you feel comfortable reporting to about your fitness efforts. Consider family members and close friends that might be willing to work with you in your efforts to get physically *fit for good*. On the lines below, write the names of three people who come to mind.

1. _____
2. _____
3. _____

Now act. Prayerfully select an individual who you think would be the best fit as your fitness fellow—the person that you will return and report to on your efforts to exercise according to your fitness focus. Share with them your understanding of the eternal marks, the sweat, and the fiery darts, and share your desire to experiment upon the Word of God according to His pattern of creation. Share your fitness focus and then invite him or her to be your fitness fellow to help you claim the blessings of each phase of the Creation in the following chapters. If the individual accepts your invitation, explain to him or her what the position entails and have your fitness fellow sign his or her name at the bottom right of your fitness sphere. If not, return to your list and pick another individual who you feel would be a better fit to be your fitness fellow.

In addition to a fitness fellow, you'll need a mentor—the perfect mentor, Jesus Christ.

"He who is our Great Redeemer was fully qualified to become such, because He was and is the Great Emulator! We, in turn, have been asked to emulate Him."[6]

In my life, living through the pain of losing a brother to suicide, healing through grief, rebuilding myself after a failed business, walking through the darkness after a miscarriage and postpartum depression, surviving a rocky marriage, living away from my husband for many years due to his

Create a Fitness Focus

military service, being broke, struggling to raise small kids, and moving every two years, I am no stranger to sadness and pain.

In all my struggles, I always knew to look to those who could show me a better way—to look for someone who had been successful in what I wanted to do or who I wanted to become. After saving my marriage, healing my grief and sadness, rebuilding a business, and creating a new relationship with my Heavenly Father, my Savior, and the Spirit, I decided to become a life coach for women.

I once had a client tell me that she wished she could keep me in her pocket at all times. She needed someone there to redirect her, guide her, and help her on her way. Another client, around the same time, expressed to me how she wished I could take the pain away. Back then I just taught self-control principles—generic habits and rituals. I soon became very frustrated that I couldn't help people more. I went to my Heavenly Father in prayer. I expressed to Him how I wanted to be able to save my clients.

This time in prayer led to an amazing life-changing experience with my Heavenly Father and the Spirit. I was taught my role and my assignment in helping my clients and the sisters I would meet around the world. My perspective shifted as I realized that my assignment is to lead people to the great Mentor and to refer people to the great Counselor. From that point on, I was freed from the pressure to redirect people in their choices for self-control and started redirecting people to self-mastery (see Chapter 9). *Mastery* requires a master. It requires a change of heart. It requires humility.

> We can change our behavior. Our very desires can change. How? There is only one way. True change—permanent change—can come only through the healing, cleansing, and enabling power of the Atonement of Jesus Christ. He loves you—each of you! He allows you to access His power as you keep His commandments, eagerly, earnestly, and exactly. It is that simple and certain. The gospel of Jesus Christ *is* a gospel of change!
>
> A strong human spirit with control over appetites of the flesh is master over emotions and passions and not a slave to them. That kind of freedom is as vital to the spirit as oxygen is to the body! Freedom from self-slavery is true liberation!"[7]

Fit for Good

Having a body and living in this physical world gives us the ultimate opportunity to learn self-mastery. Becoming *fit for good* is taking you on the same path you are taking to become like the Master. It is not about manipulation or control—it is actually about using our agency to be humble and have a change of heart.

To get the best results for fitness success, these are the principles I use and require when someone works with me in my programs:

1. Humility—being open and coachable
2. Honesty—allowing me to know all the details to help me create a plan of action based on real, accurate data
3. Accountability—Willingness to be held accountable.

When I look at the things I require from my clients, I am in awe of the eternal pattern that the Savior uses as my Mentor—a pattern He can use with you too. Approaching our Heavenly Father in true humility is the fastest way to start receiving answers to prayers. When we approach our Heavenly Father with a humble heart, we demonstrate to Him that we are open to His ideas. If we act as if He is a genie in a bottle that we can make petitions to and He will grant our every wish, we will not truly change our behaviors. Being honest with God is probably one of the hardest things for me to do. I believe it is because we have to get real with ourselves. This process is uncomfortable.

Willingness to be held accountable is the clincher to lasting success when working with a mentor. When we are learning and growing, we are stretched to a new capacity of strength. Our willingness to stretch and trust in faith is foundational when we work with the great Mentor.

The best mentors care about your success, love you, and will hold you to a new line to help you stretch and learn. Especially expect this from the great Mentor, Jesus Christ. He loves you and wants your success, but as you grow and learn to emulate Him, you *will* be stretched to reach the capacity of greatness that is in you.

In this process of tutoring and mentoring, you will quickly discover that chastening is involved both in the Lord's questions and in His training

Create a Fitness Focus

of us. The Lord tells us that He chastens those whom He loves. In fact, the chastened may be the only individuals willing to learn (see Mosiah 23:21). After all, where could one get more profound, personal insights than from the Lord and in the context of divine charity?

With a fitness focus statement, Fitness Focus Sphere, a fitness fellow, and the perfect Mentor, you are ready to return and report on your efforts to form, divide, beautify, and multiply your physical capacity to fill the measure of your creation with a fulness of joy.

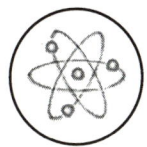

Create a *fitness focus statement*. Select a *fitness fellow* to return and report to about your efforts to claim the blessings of exercising according to the Lord's pattern of creation.

LINE UPON LINE SUMMARY

On Your Mark

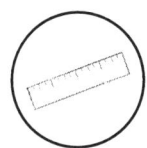 Receive God's image. Remember, your body is *the measure of your creation*—the physical manifestation of your potential to become like God.

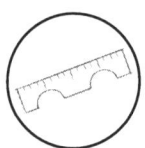 Yoke yourself to Christ when you exercise. Remember, *His yoke will enable* the measure of your creation to be filled with a fulness of joy.

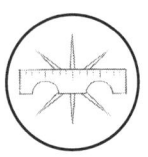 Invite the Spirit to be with you when you exercise. Remember, *His power will quicken* the measure of your creation so you can experience a fulness of joy.

Create a Fitness Focus

LINE UPON LINE SUMMARY

Get Set

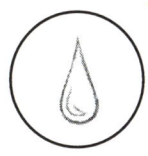 Sweat in the wilderness of regular exercise. The *sweat of your brow* is the manifestation of your effort to subject the fallen elements of your body to your divine spirit.

 Defend against the adversary's fiery darts. *Watch and pray* for protection against the darts of physical lust, latency, and limits that will fill the measure of your creation with misery.

 Experiment upon the word of God. By *exercising faith in the word of God*, you can increase your physical capacity to fill the measure of your creation with a fulness of joy.

LINE UPON LINE SUMMARY

Go!

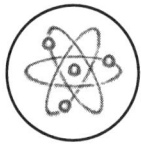

Create a *fitness focus statement*. Select a *fitness fellow* to return and report to about your efforts to claim the blessings of exercising according to the Lord's pattern of creation.

CHAPTER 8

Form Your Flesh

"If you go, I'll go," said my father, tipping the scale in his favor. My mother couldn't pass up the opportunity. They exited the large pool and headed toward the three-meter springboard at the Glenwood Hot Springs Pool in Colorado. My father had made the deal so that he and the large crowd at the pool could watch my mother, a former competitive diver at Ricks College (now known as Brigham Young University–Idaho), dive. As a gentleman should, my father insisted that my mother go first. She wouldn't have it any other way because this way she could see him dive after her. She climbed up the ladder and faced the pool. Instinctively, she paused to gather her thoughts. It had been a few years since she had attempted such a dive.

My father recalls that as soon as she stepped on the springboard, many of the about one hundred swimmers took notice of this attractive young lady preparing to dive. My mother exhaled and gracefully stepped forward to the end of the board. After turning her back to the water, she stepped off her approach. The precision of her movements intrigued and increased the spectators. They knew they were about to witness an impressive dive. My mother turned to face the water, stepped forward, and launched herself upward with both arms above her head and a sharp single leg. She landed gracefully on the end of the springboard as it gave way to the perfection of her *form*. The board forcefully recoiled and sent her soaring upward. At the peak of her ascent, she gracefully piked forward and touched her toes. During her descent, she opened her *form,* and with extended arms and pointed toes, she sliced through the water. She surfaced and then swam to the shallow end of the large pool. She stood and faced my father, waved her hand, and signaled with a smile that it was his turn.

After watching such a beautiful dive, the majority of the swimmers were now focused on my father. He confidently ascended the ladder. My father presented an impressive physique thanks to his habit of doing push-ups each morning. He stood near the end of the diving board to gather his jumbled thoughts. *I must do exactly what Kitty did,* he said to himself as he walked to the end of the board. He turned around and stepped off his approach in exactly the same manner as my mother. Now every swimmer seemed to be watching my father. My mother said she could feel the excitement of the crowd. This muscular diver was about to unleash a dive unlike any they had seen before. My father did not disappoint. He stepped forward and leaped upward with both arms above his head and a sharp single leg. He landed powerfully on the end of the springboard. It groaned under his muscular momentum, but then quickly recoiled, launching my father upward more forcefully than he had expected.

From the moment my father's feet left the board, his *form* failed. He began to flail his arms and legs in an attempt to stay upright. Surprisingly, at the peak of his ascent, he tried to apply the pike position. My mother recalls that at that moment my father looked very much like a stinkbug in his bent position. As he was dropping, my father realized that if he opened up from his position, he would land parallel to the water and experience a monumental and painful belly flop. So my father stuck with his stinkbug position to the bitter end. He hit the water with a thunderous WHOPP!

My mother cringed at the sound. She and the other spectators waited for my father to surface. A few bubbles rippled to the top, but no sign of my father. The tension began to build as the water continued to settle. There was still no sign of my father. My mother's heart began to sink

Form Your Flesh

as she thought the worst. She began to step toward the deep end of the pool when she caught a glimpse of a swimmer, a very muscular swimmer, struggling to swim under the water toward her. Suddenly, like a whale breaching the water in the wild, my father came up out of the water gasping for air. He had swum under the water all the way from his point of entry hoping that he could escape the embarrassment of his failed dive. My mother relaxed and smiled as she walked toward the panting love of her life.

The difference between my mother's and father's dives was their *form*. My mother had the physical capacity to form her body for the dive because she had several years of practice. My father had the physical capacity to do a hundred push-ups, but not a dive (though I'm sure those push-ups helped him courageously accept and survive the impact of his failed dive).

FORM

In the first phase of the Creation, the Lord exercised dominion over the elements of the universe to *form* the earth (see Abraham 4:1), to provide a *physical place* for His children to receive the experiences and blessings that would allow them to fill the measure of their creation with joy (see Abraham 3:24). He formed the waters, the dry land, "every herb yielding seed," and "every living creature that moveth" (Moses 2:12, 21; see also Moses 2:9–27) to provide a place for His children to dwell (see Abraham 3:24).

In exercising, this phase of the Creation can be likened to the measure of joy that comes from forming our flesh. The desire for this type of joy is the primary driving force behind today's fitness industry. It is the joy of before-and-after pictures, the joy of sensual strolls down the beach in slimming summer swimsuits. However, like summer itself, the joy found in this phase will *diminish* and give way to fall, and eventually to the Fall of Adam, as our bodies return to the dust from which they were made (see Genesis 3:19).

When the element of time is added to each quadrant of the matrix, the measure of joy experienced in each quadrant is revealed. As shown below, the joy we *get* from impressing *others* with our physical form in the first quadrant will *diminish* over time as the elements of our bodies succumb to the wrinkles and wounds of mortality.

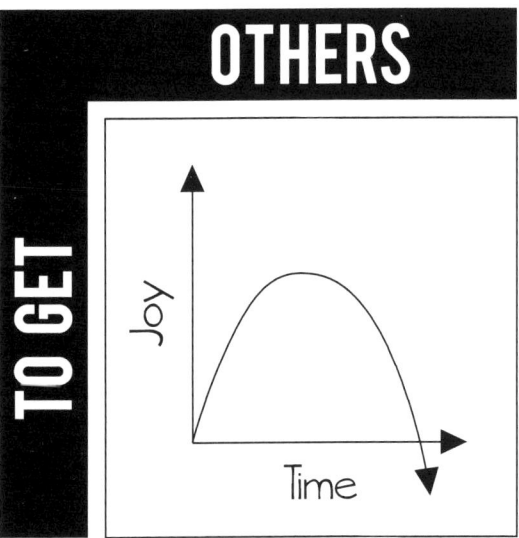

The adversary knows that our joy in this phase can't last. He will hurl his fiery darts to ignite the carnal kerosene of our fallen natures and keep us addicted to, condemned by, and comatose in this phase of the Creation. He does this by enticing us to partake of his lustful liquors of body worship, loathing, and apathy.

The most propagandized and consumed liquor of the three is the sweet wine of body worship—the addictive liquor that fuels the fashion, sex, body piercing, and tattoo industries. We taste it when we exercise to *form* our flesh for the bursts of pleasure that come from the compliment of a friend, the lustful glance or gawk of a stranger, or from acceptance into high society's circle of perceived physical perfection. Satan serves his lustful liquor from pints of pride in the upper dining halls of the "great and spacious building" (1 Nephi 8:31). When our fitness efforts are focused on filling the measure of our creation with the sweetness of this wine, we run the risk of becoming "lovers of pleasures more than lovers of God; having a *form* of godliness, but *denying* the power thereof" (2 Timothy 3:4–5; emphasis added).

Form Your Flesh

Body loathing is the bitter beer of physical self-hate. Satan brews it in the vats of mental, physical, and emotional abuse. He serves it in the condemned lower and lonely bars of the great and spacious building, and we drink it whenever we find fault in or have hate toward our physical *form*. We consume it when we hide in our homes and virtual realities to protect ourselves from self-hate and to dull its pain.

The reckless rum of body apathy is the most deadly of the three. Satan serves it from a "shot" on the upper floors of the great and spacious building. It causes a comatose state in which we "neglect" and "take no thought for [the] nourishment" and care of our physical *form* (Alma 32:38). This liquor leads both the couch potato and the extreme thrill seeker to cast the pearl of their body before the swine of indulgence. Body apathy can cut life short either because of the couch potato's morbidity or the thrill seeker's mortality.

In order to remain "sober" (Alma 38:15) and free from the influence of these liquors, you must seek for the blessing that will increase your physical capacity to fulfill your fitness focus rather than the *diminishing* joy that is found in this phase.

GO!

One Sunday while passing between sacrament meeting and Sunday School, I witnessed a sobering moment that helped me understand the blessing of this phase. A visiting and very precocious little girl walked up to a sweet sister in our ward and asked, "Why are you so big?" My heart dropped. I turned instinctively toward the child to save this sister from the embarrassment of answering her question. But before I could snatch her, this sister crouched over, placed her hands on her knees, looked intently into the little girl's eyes, and said with a soft voice, "I am big so I can give big hugs." The girl smiled and leaped into her open arms.

In that moment, that wonderful sister taught me that our physical form, no matter its shape, size, or color, has one purpose—every element in your body, from the tip of your longest toe to the crown of your head, functions so you can *act* to fill the measure of your creation with joy.

The divine blessing that comes from forming our flesh is an *increased physical capacity to act,* or in other words, physical fitness. Over the last several decades, the medical world has created various ways to assess an individual's physical fitness. One of the most commonly known measurements is the Body Mass Index (BMI). Medical and fitness professionals use the BMI to measure the mass of a person's body in relation to his or her height and weight. Professionals use it as a tool to measure an individual's risk of disease. Remember that sweet sister in the church hallway? She taught me that the BMI can be used to measure so much more.

See the basic BMI chart for adults on the opposite page.

Examine the chart, and mark your BMI by marking where your current height (left side) and weight in pounds (right side) intersect on the chart. Watch out! Don't down a shot of body apathy by not taking the time to mark the chart. Don't drink the bitter beer of body loathing if your mark lands in the obese or overweight range of the chart. Don't sip the wine of body worship if your mark fits "perfectly" into the healthy weight range.

"Be sober" (1 Peter 5:8) by remembering the sister in the hallway—your mark has absolutely *nothing* to do with your self-worth and *everything* to do with your physical capacity to act. The BMI is a measurement of how much energy is in your body; it is a measurement of Body Mass *Investment* rather than just an index of your risk for disease. Therefore, if your mark landed on the left side of the chart, know this: your body is ready to receive more energy so you can act to fill the measure of your creation with joy. If your mark landed on the right side, know this: your body is full of potential energy ready to fuel your efforts to fill the measure of your creation with joy.

The same type of thinking can help with other health measurements that may lead to body loathing—health measurements like high blood pressure, high cholesterol, and high glucose levels. You can view all of those measurements as a witness of your body's efforts to provide you with the blood pressure, materials, and instant energy to act to fill the measure

Body Mass Index (BMI) Table
(Adult Men & Women)

	Underweight				Normal							Overweight						Obese				
BMI	16	17	18	19	20	21	22	23	24	25	26	27	28	29	30	31	32	33	34	35
Height									Body Weight (pounds)											
4'10"	77	82	86	91	96	100	105	110	115	119	124	129	134	138	143	148	153	158	162	167
4'11"	79	84	89	94	99	104	109	114	119	124	128	133	138	143	148	153	158	163	168	173
5'	82	87	92	97	102	107	112	118	123	128	133	138	143	148	153	158	163	168	174	179
5'1"	85	90	96	100	106	111	116	122	127	132	137	143	148	153	158	164	169	174	180	185
5'2"	88	93	99	104	109	115	120	126	131	136	142	147	153	158	164	169	175	180	186	191
5'3"	91	96	102	107	113	118	124	130	135	141	146	152	158	163	169	175	180	186	191	197
5'4"	93	99	105	110	116	122	128	134	140	145	151	157	163	169	174	180	186	192	197	204
5'5"	96	102	108	114	120	126	132	138	144	150	156	162	168	174	180	186	192	198	204	210
5'6"	99	106	112	118	124	130	136	142	148	155	161	167	173	179	186	192	198	204	210	216
5'7"	102	109	115	121	127	134	140	146	153	159	166	172	178	185	191	198	204	211	217	223
5'8"	105	112	119	125	131	138	144	151	158	164	171	177	184	190	197	203	210	216	223	230
5'9"	109	115	122	128	135	142	149	155	162	169	176	182	189	196	203	209	216	223	230	236
5'10"	112	119	126	132	139	146	153	160	167	174	181	188	195	202	209	216	222	229	236	243
5'11"	115	122	129	136	143	150	157	165	172	179	186	193	200	208	215	222	229	236	243	250
6'	118	125	133	140	147	154	162	169	177	184	191	199	206	213	221	228	235	242	250	258
6'1"	121	129	137	144	151	159	166	174	182	189	197	204	212	219	227	235	242	250	257	265
6'2"	125	133	140	148	155	163	171	179	186	194	202	210	218	225	233	241	249	256	264	272
6'3"	128	136	144	152	160	168	176	184	192	200	208	216	224	232	240	248	256	264	272	279

Source: Adapted from *Clinical Guidelines on the Identification, Evaluation, and Treatment of Overweight and Obesity in Adults*, 1998.

of your creation with joy. You simply need to act in a manner that will maximize those efforts.

I shared this idea with a dear friend recently. I will call her Shelley to maintain privacy. Shelley wasn't her chipper self during her physical therapy exam. I had gotten to know her better as I worked closely with her to alleviate her lower back pain, so I could tell that something was eating at her.

"Are you doing okay?" I asked.

"Yeah, I'm okay. I'm just feeling a little down today," she responded, as she sat on the exam table.

"Why?" I asked.

"To tell you the truth, I stepped on the scale this morning, and I'm way overweight! I've never weighed this much in my life," she replied in despair.

I followed up with a few questions about her weight gain and then asked if I could help her form a new idea about weight gain. With her permission, I shared with her the lesson I had learned from that sister in the hallway at church. Shelley later shared with me her thoughts about that lesson. Here are her words:

> When I went to physical therapy that day, I was feeling discouraged about my current health and recent weight gain. I knew that I had gained weight since the previous physical therapy session a year earlier. I had been feeling particularly frustrated at my extra weight and admitted my guilt. Weight had not been an issue in my life until the past few years due to health struggles and probably contributing age factors. But [Rich's] response was not what I had expected to hear. With concern and kindness, [he] shared with me [his] thoughts about what weight gain really was. As I listened, I began to feel uplifted. I realized my extra pounds were not meant to be heavy on my spirit. My extra weight could be used as extra energy of love that I could give away to others. I realized that by accepting myself, I had more to give physically to the Lord and others around me. It was a reminder of who I am in the Lord's eyes and who I can become. I left my appointment feeling lighter, spiritually and physically! It was the brightness of hope I had been seeking.
>
> When I got out to my car, I said a little prayer. I thanked my Heavenly Father that I had been reminded of who I can truly become.

Form Your Flesh

> Afterward, I felt so enlightened that I went and visited my husband at work. I shared my experience with him. This extra weight gain and physical challenges were not meant to discourage me but to inspire me to seek out what Heavenly Father would like me to do to improve my physical state. This in turn has led me to start an exercise program that has helped me feel better for all the *right* reasons. I learned through this experience that my health and weight need to be in accordance with what I need to accomplish for the Lord. When I exercise with this in mind, I take on a new level of commitment and dedication. I am content in knowing my potential can be attained when I spiritually work with my physical state.

Shelley had sobered up and saw her weight gain as it really was—not as a measurement of her self-worth, but as a physical witness of her physical potential to bless the lives of those she loved.

You can do the same and claim the blessing of this phase by measuring and reporting on your efforts to increase your physical capacity to fulfill your fitness focus. I recommend using a simple comprehensive assessment of five various physical measurements—standing reach, tightrope walk, sit-to-stand, push-ups, and BMI, to report on your physical capacity to act. This assessment, called the Capacity to Act Score, tests your flexibility, balance, endurance, strength, and body composition in less than five minutes. In order to calculate your score, you will need a stopwatch, a tape measure, a sturdy chair, a scale, and your fitness fellow to measure and record your scores in the box below.

Fit for Good

Capacity to Act Score	
Activity	Score
Sit-to-Stand	
Tightrope Walk	
Push-ups	
Standing Reach	
BMI	
Capacity to Act Score	

You will spend the first minute of the test measuring your lower extremity strength and endurance. Sit in a sturdy chair. Cross your arms against your chest and have your fitness fellow count how many times you can stand up and sit down in one minute. To ensure a full sit-to-stand repetition, make sure you lift both feet slightly off the ground before you stand up and that your knees fully extend when you stand.

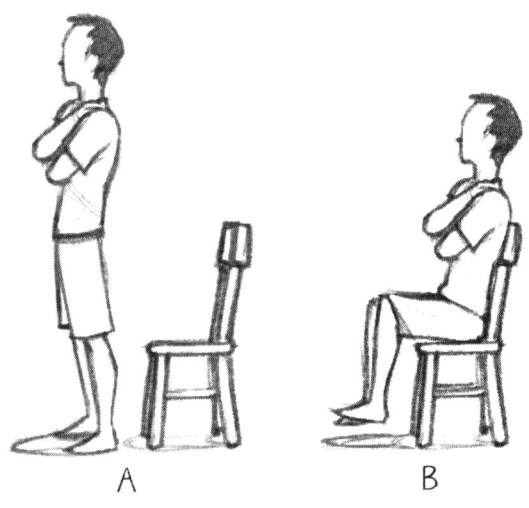

A   B

Form Your Flesh

Record your score based on the following standards:

- 0–4 reps = 1 point
- 5–9 reps = 2 points
- 10–14 reps = 3 points
- 15–19 reps = 4 points
- 20–24 reps = 5 points
- 25–29 reps = 6 points
- 30–34 reps = 7 points
- 35–39 reps = 8 points
- 40–44 reps = 9 points
- 45–50 reps = 10 points
- 50+ reps = additional 1 point per sit-to-stand over 50

The second activity, the tightrope walk, will assess your balance. Stand with your arms crossed over your chest. Now place the heel of one foot in front of the other as if you are walking on a tightrope. If you are under fifty years old and in good health, complete the test with your eyes closed. Have your fitness fellow count how many steps in a row you take before you lose your balance.

Record your score by giving yourself a point for each step you take in a row, up to 10 points.

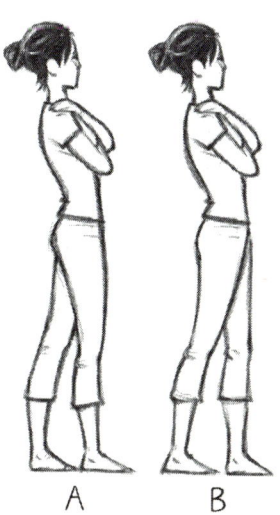

A   B

Fit for Good

The third activity, push-ups, will take one minute to complete. This activity will measure your upper-body strength and endurance. Start by lying facedown on the ground and place your hands at a distance that is slightly wider then shoulder-width apart, with your shoulders, hips, and heels in a straight line. It helps to mentally tighten your buttocks and abdominals to help line up your body. Look straight ahead as you extend your elbows to push your body up. Complete one push-up repetition by lowering your body until your elbows are flexed at a 90 degree angle. The test is stopped as soon as your knees touch the ground or at the end of the sixty seconds, whichever comes first.

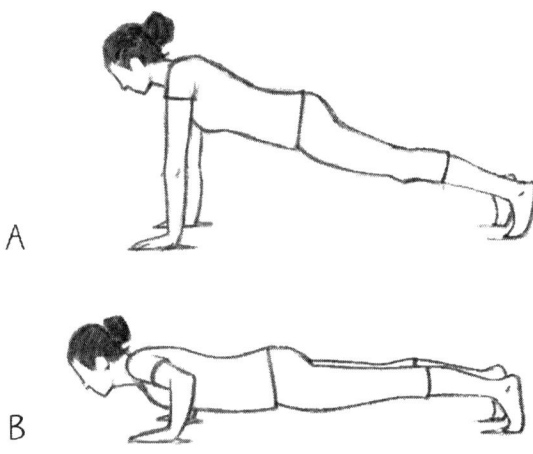

Have your fitness fellow count how many push-ups you can do in one minute. (If you are physically unable to perform floor push-ups then replace them with wall push-ups). Score yourself based on the following standards:

- 1–5 reps = 1 point
- 6–10 reps = 2 points
- 11–15 reps = 3 points
- 16–20 reps = 4 points

- 21–24 reps = 5 points
- 25–27 reps = 6 points
- 28–29 reps = 7 points
- 30–31 reps = 8 points
- 32–33 reps = 9 points
- 34–35 reps = 10 points
- 35+ reps = additional 1 point per push-up over 35

Rest for thirty seconds as your fitness fellow marks your score in your chart.

The fourth activity will measure your standing flexibility. Stand with your feet facing forward and shoulder-width apart. While keeping your knees straight, reach down with both arms toward the floor.

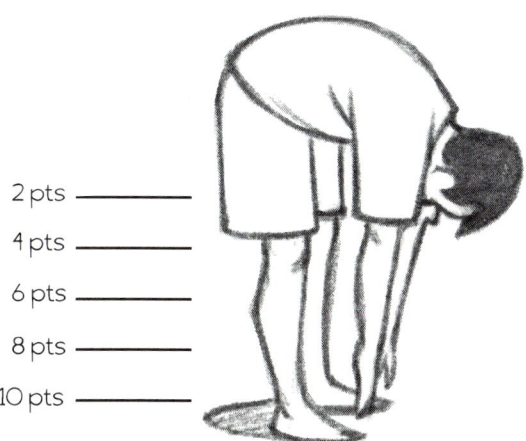

Record your score based on the following standards:
- Touch your mid-thighs = 2 points
- Touch your knees = 4 points
- Touch your mid-shins = 6 points
- Touch your ankles = 8 points
- Touch your toes = 10 points

Fit for Good

The last test, the BMI, will measure your body composition. Use the BMI you calculated earlier to score yourself according to the following standards:

- BMI greater than 45 or less than 13 = 1 point
- BMI from 41 to 45 or 13 to 14 = 2 points
- BMI from 36 to 40 or 14 to 15 = 4 points
- BMI from 31 to 35 or 15 to 16 = 6 points
- BMI from 26 to 30 or 17 to 18 = 8 points
- BMI from 18 to 25 = 10 points

Remember, this is your Body Mass *Investment* score. If your BMI is high, your body is full of potential energy ready to be used. If your BMI is low, your body is ready to receive more energy.

Calculate your Capacity to Act Score by totaling your points and putting that total at the bottom of the chart. The higher your score, the greater your current physical capacity to act can be.

Now lay claim to the blessing of this phase of the Creation. Exercise not to receive the diminishing joy that comes from impressing others with your physical form but to increase your physical capacity to act. Record your initial Capacity to Act Score at the top of your Fitness Focus Sphere, and at the end of your four-week cycle, retest to measure your increased physical capacity to act.

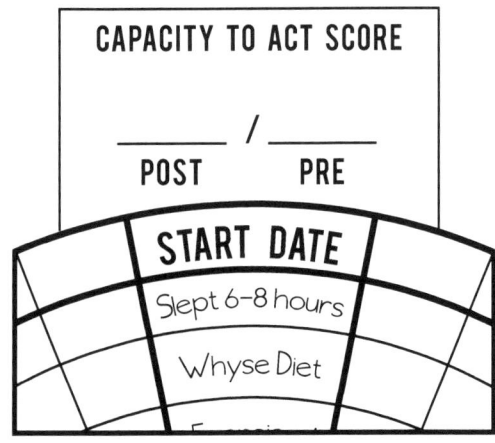

Form Your Flesh

Remember, because of the Savior's Atonement, you are "free according to the flesh" to form your flesh to increase your physical capacity to participate in the fourth phase of the Creation, or to form your flesh "according to the captivity and power of the devil" by becoming addicted to, condemned by, or comatose in this phase of the Creation (2 Nephi 2:27). As you measure and report on your efforts to *form* your body to increase your physical capacity to act, you will be ready to claim the blessing of the second phase of the Creation. The second phase will help you *divide* the light from the darkness within, and increase your physical capacity to fill the measure of your creation with a fulness of joy.

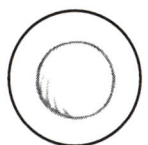

Form your flesh by exercising to *increase your physical capacity to act.*

LINE UPON LINE SUMMARY

On Your Mark

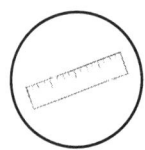 Receive God's image. Remember, your body is *the measure of your creation*—the physical manifestation of your potential to become like God.

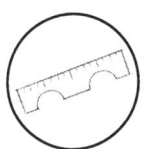 Yoke yourself to Christ when you exercise. Remember, *His yoke will enable* the measure of your creation to be filled with a fulness of joy.

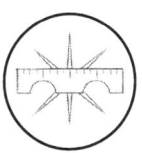 Invite the Spirit to be with you when you exercise. Remember, *His power will quicken* the measure of your creation so you can experience a fulness of joy.

Form Your Flesh

LINE UPON LINE SUMMARY

Get Set

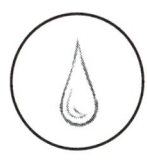
Sweat in the wilderness of regular exercise. The *sweat of your brow* is the manifestation of your effort to subject the fallen elements of your body to your divine spirit.

Defend against the adversary's fiery darts. *Watch and pray* for protection against the darts of physical lust, latency, and limits that will fill the measure of your creation with misery.

Experiment upon the word of God. By *exercising faith in the word of God*, you can increase your physical capacity to fill the measure of your creation with a fulness of joy.

LINE UPON LINE SUMMARY

Go!

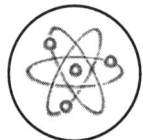

Create a *fitness focus statement*. Select a *fitness fellow* to return and report to about your efforts to claim the blessings of exercising according to the Lord's pattern of creation.

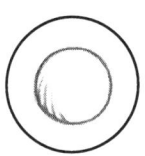

Form your flesh by exercising to *increase your physical capacity to act*.

CHAPTER 9

Divide the Light from the Darkness Within

I had never before experienced such deep darkness. Because I spent my childhood living in the bright light of Arizona, I found the darkness overwhelming. I felt like I had been plunged into a pool of thick blackness that seemed to creep into me and constrict every part and function of my body.

This darkness came from deep below the Blue Mountains near Sydney, Australia. After I graduated from high school, my Arizona high school football team was invited to play a game of football against a local team in Australia. As part of our trip, we took a tour of a large cavern thousands of feet below the mountains. Once we were settled in the cavern, our tour guide began to share with us the history of the cave. I vividly remember his description of how the aborigines of that area would use the cavern to punish those who had committed serious crimes against the tribe. They would escort them to the cavern and leave them in its darkness. He related that they would live for only a short period of time. They would die either by hurling themselves over an unseen cliff or by sending their body into shock because of hallucinations induced by the darkness.

To give us a small taste of the complete absence of light in the cave, our guide informed us that he would soon turn off the cavern lights and let our eyes adjust to the complete darkness. He would then have us stand still for what he said would feel like the longest minute of our lives. He invited us to find a safe place to stand and then proceeded to turn off the cavern lights. Instantly, a thick blackness engulfed us as every particle of light fled the cavern. Small gasps and whimpers of anxiousness echoed through the cavern as our bodies tried to adjust to the stifling darkness. The guide then asked us to see if we could see our hands in front of our faces. Absolutely nothing was visible. He then asked us to remain silent and still. *Beep*! The start of the tour guide's stopwatch pierced the cavern air.

The complete darkness seemed to slow time. My thoughts began to turn toward my family. I recalled my parents sending me off to Australia from the airport in Arizona. I thought about my recent graduation from high school and the graduation gift my parents had given me, a wristwatch that had the latest Indigo backlight technology. The temptation was too great. I grabbed for my watch and pressed the backlight button—*letting* a beam of blue light pierce the darkness of the cavern. After two or three seconds, the light quickly faded away. I pressed it again. The light caused one of my teammates to come toward me and ask, "What is that?" I told him about my watch and then pressed the backlight again and again. Our minute of darkness concluded as the guide turned the cavern lights on. I was surprised to see several of my teammates huddled around me. They were *physically* drawn to the dividing light of my watch.

DIVIDE

In the second phase of the Earth's creation, the Lord divided the light from the darkness.

> And the earth, after it was formed, was empty and desolate, because they had not formed anything but the earth; and darkness reigned upon the face of the deep, and the Spirit of the Gods was brooding upon the face of the waters. And they (the Gods) said: *Let* there be light; and there was light. And they (the Gods) comprehended the light, for it was bright; and they divided the light, or *caused* it to be *divided*, from the darkness. (Abraham 4:2–4; emphasis added)

Divide the Light from the Darkness Within

Take notice of the Lord's pattern in that scripture. He first *let* there be light, and then he *caused*, or controlled, the division of the light from the darkness. This divine pattern of *letting* there be light and *causing* it to be divided from the darkness is the pattern that will enable you to claim the blessing of the second phase of the Creation.

Many people participate in this phase to experience the joy of *getting*, or gaining, more control over the elements of their bodies for *themselves*. This phase can motivate you to exercise to get control of your blood pressure, to "own" the flight of stairs at work, to run a 10 km race in less than an hour, or to conquer the switchbacks of the Grand Canyon. The joy of gaining control for yourself will continue to increase as long as you gain *more* control over your blood pressure, "own" a *more* challenging flight of stairs, run a *faster* time in a 10 km race, or find a *more* "grand" canyon to conquer. As depicted in the graph below, your joy will be *limited* over time because you can lower your blood pressure only so low, climb only so many stairs, run a 10 km race only so fast, and climb only so many switchbacks.

The adversary knows that, over time, this phase can bring you only limited joy. He will use his fiery darts to keep you damned in this phase by tempting you to act in a manner that will limit your physical capacity

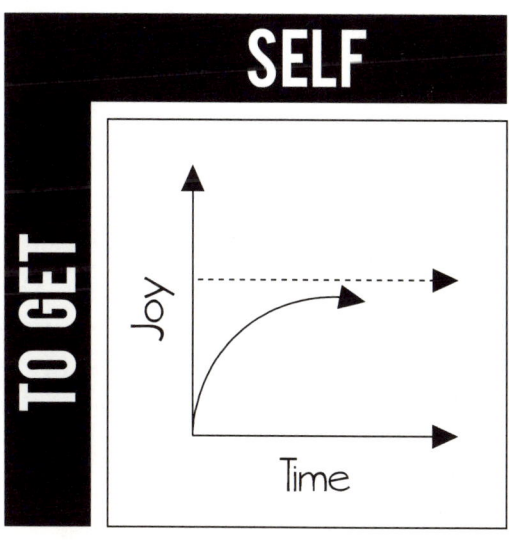

to exercise dominion over the elements of your body altogether, or by tempting you to become *obsessed* with the desire to gain more and more control over the elements of your body.

There are two prominent tactics the devil will use to tempt you to limit your physical capacity to exercise dominion over the elements of your body. The first happens when Satan blurs the physical line that the Lord drew when He divided the light from the darkness in the Creation—creating day and night (see Moses 2:4–5). The world's continuous and instant access to almost everything has dulled this division, giving people "more" time to work and play in the dark hours of the night. He knows that when you work or play in these dark hours, your capacity to claim the blessing of this phase is limited because of the fatigue-based fuel and cover of the night that these hours provide for the natural man within you.

The second tactic that he employs is the temptation to partake of food as a substance to abuse rather than as sustenance that sustains life. He inscribes this abuse in his culinary calling card to eat and drink to "be merry" (see 2 Nephi 28:7). I am not suggesting that the comfort and merriment that can come from drinking and eating food is inherently evil; I love Thanksgiving dinner! However, I am suggesting that the addictive and comatose consumption of food is a powerful tool that the adversary uses to limit our capacity to exercise faith. Remember, in chapter 6 we learned that faith "is the *moving cause of all action, in them*; that *without it, both mind and body would be in a state of inactivity*, and all their exertions would cease, both physical and mental."[1] The adversary knows this and will tempt us to overeat and to overwhelm our bodies with so much extra energy that our physical capacity to exercise the faith that will fill the measure of our creations with joy will be limited. For example, overeating can limit our ability to experience the simple and sweet joys of life, such as playing a ball game with your children or grandchildren in the backyard. Overeating can also limit your ability to experience the more profound joys of life, such as accepting the call to serve a mission.

If the previous tactics fail, the adversary will often flip his approach, and instead of using temptations that will limit our capacity to control

Divide the Light from the Darkness Within

our bodies, he tempts us to become addicted to the pleasure that comes from gaining more and more control over the elements of our bodies. This obsession develops when we succumb to his temptation to lose ten *more* pounds, run a *faster* 10 km race, and conquer *more* of the Grand Canyon to keep us from claiming the blessings of the next phases. Remember that your quest for more control will always be limited by the gravity of your fallen physical state.

Once again, the key to defend against the adversary's fiery darts is that instead of focusing on the *limited* joy of this phase, focus on claiming the blessing of this phase that will increase your physical capacity to fulfill your fitness focus.

GO!

We claim the blessing of this phase when we follow the Lord's example by physically "[letting] there be light" in our lives and then causing it to be "divided . . . from the darkness" within us (Moses 2:3–4).

The thought of physically "letting there be light" in our lives may seem foreign due to our "being in the dark" when it comes to understanding what light is. In physics, light is the energy of creation. It is the material that all mass is made of, and it is the energy that enables all mass to transform from one state to another. In the gospel, Mormon defined light primarily as the influence of Christ that enables man to know right from wrong (see Moroni 7:16). In section 88 of the Doctrine and Covenants, the Lord deepens our understanding of physical light and gospel light, bringing those two concepts and their beauty together:

> This is the light of Christ. As also he is in the sun, and *the light of the sun*, and *the power* thereof by which it was made. . . .
>
> And the light which shineth, which giveth you light, is through him who enlighteneth your eyes, *which is the same light* that quickeneth your understandings;
>
> Which light proceedeth forth from the presence of God to fill the immensity of space—The light which is in all things, *which giveth life to all things* (D&C 88:7, 11–13; emphasis added).

Take a moment and let the light of these scriptures "enlighten" your mind. Can you see the connection? The physical light that comes from the sun *is* the light of Christ! It *is* His light that both enlightens your eyes to see and enlightens your mind to understand the mysteries of God. It *is* His light that is in all things, that gives life to all things—the very light that pulses within your brain and throughout your body, giving life to every particle of your physical being. All light is His Light!

When we physically *let* His light into our lives, we can claim the blessing of this phase—*the increased physical capacity to practice* not self-control, but *self-mastery*, which will cause the light to be divided from the darkness of the natural man within us.

The difference between self-control and self-mastery is found in the power source they draw upon. Self-control draws upon the power of one's own will. Self-mastery draws upon the enabling power of the Master (see Ether 12:27). We can increase our physical capacity to practice self-mastery by physically letting the enabling light of the Master into our lives.

The Savior has revealed three practices that will physically let His light into our lives. The first practice is a direct derivative of the Lord's divine division that created night and day. The divine division is found in the Lord's command that we "retire to [our] bed early, that [we] may not be weary; arise early, that [our] bodies and [our] minds may be invigorated" (D&C 88:124). The Lord commands us to partake of His divine and dividing gift of sleep.

Scientists are still uncertain as to why we sleep. However, several theories have been developed that, when viewed under the light of the restored gospel, help us recognize how this divine gift lets Christ's light into our lives. According to the Harvard Medical School Division of Sleep Medicine, one of the earliest theories suggested that sleep serves as a "survival function," protecting us during the dark hours of the night, a time when we are "particularly vulnerable" to predators.[2] Another more recent theory suggests that sleep provides the body with an opportunity to repair the wear and tear and remove the toxins that develop during the day.

Divide the Light from the Darkness Within

The most recent theory suggests that sleep serves as the time in which the brain actually downloads the previous day's experiences into its hard memory to be used to improve the efficiency and performance of the body the next day. In short, these theories define sleep as a state and place of personal protection, restoration, and edification.

When viewed under the Master's light, sleep becomes a time in which we are blessed to physically enter into the "rest of the Lord" (see Alma 16:16–17). When we "lie down unto the Lord" and divide our days with sufficient sleep each night, the Lord will "watch over [us]" (Alma 37:37). While under His watch, His light will endow us with *protection* by "putting to rest" the natural man that thrives when we are physically fatigued—think of the last time you crossed paths with a sleep-deprived toddler or teenager—and that thrives under the cover of the dark and late hours of the night. Under our Master's watch, His light will endow us with a physical *renewal* of our bodies, repairing the injuries and insults our bodies experienced during the day. His light will endow us with the *edification* of our minds. Giving our minds the time to rest and process the mental stress of the past will give us the mental capacity to function better in the future. Sleep, a continuous seven to nine hours for adults and nine to eleven hours for children,[3] is a daily and divine practice that will physically let the light of the Lord into our lives and increase our physical capacity to practice self-mastery.

The second practice that will physically let Christ's light into our lives is found in "the *order* and *will* of God in the temporal salvation of all saints in the last days" (D&C 89:2; emphasis added). The *order* of the Lord's Word of Wisdom *divides* for us that which is good for our bodies and that which is not good for our bodies. However, the *will* of the Lord or, in other words, *why* He gave us commandments concerning what we should let into our bodies, isn't as well known. In section 89, we learn that the Word of Wisdom was given to warn us of the "evils and designs which do and will exist in the hearts of conspiring men in the last days" (D&C 89:4) and so "that the destroying angel shall pass by [us], as the children of Israel, and not slay [us]" (D&C 89:21). These verses reveal that the Lord's purpose for providing us with His Word of Wisdom is to protect us from the "evils and designs" of the adversary.

Now ponder this question: How does His Word of Wisdom protect us? The answer is more than just protecting us from addictive substances such as tobacco and strong or hot drinks. In His Word of Wisdom, He commands us to eat wisely, to refrain from that which He declares is not "for the body" (D&C 89:8), and to eat with "prudence and thanksgiving" (D&C 89:11). When we wisely eat that which has been "ordained" by God "for the constitution, nature, and *use* of man" (D&C 89:10; emphasis added) we are physically *letting His light* in our bodies. His light, the energy of the food ordained for us by God, is what fuels life and gives us "health in [our] navel and marrow to [our] bones." The power of His light pulses through the neurons of our brains, giving us "wisdom and great treasures of knowledge, even hidden treasures." The power of His light fuels our fitness efforts and gives us the physical capacity to "run and not be weary" and to "walk and not faint" (D&C 89:18–20). We live by the energy of His light, and we act by the energy of His light. His modern-day Word of Wisdom has given us the wisdom to physically fill our bodies with His light, giving us the increased physical capacity to practice self-mastery.

We find the third practice that will physically let His light into our life in the Lord's simple command, "Cease to be idle" (D&C 88:124). Idleness is the reserve upon which our untamed natural man's passions graze, wander, and stampede. Alma the Younger counseled his son concerning these passions, saying, "See that ye *bridle* all your passions," and then within the same verse he invited his son to "refrain from *idleness*" (Alma 38:12; emphasis added).

Ceasing to be idle can serve as a powerful bridle by which we can increase our physical capacity to practice self-mastery. In the scriptures, we have two examples of this—one positive and one negative. We find the first example in Joseph of Egypt's trial of chastity. When pitted against the sensual advancements of Potiphar's wife, Joseph quickly bridled the passions of his body by ceasing to be idle. He "fled, and got [himself] out"

Divide the Light from the Darkness Within

(Genesis 39:12). His choice to cease to be idle and to flee from a tempting situation placed him on a path of service, salvation, and joy. We find the second example in King David's trial of chastity. However, he failed to bridle his passions because he "tarried *still* at Jerusalem" (2 Samuel 11:1–4; emphasis added), a decision that allowed his natural man's passions to stampede, dragging him down a dark path of immorality, murder, and misery.

The practice of ceasing to be idle through regular physical exercise can become a powerful bridle to help you master the passions of your natural man. Do you remember Christ's forty days and forty nights in the wilderness? This wilderness experience enabled Him to subject, or bridle, the fallen elements of His mortal body to the will of His divine spirit. Daily treks into the wilderness of physical exercise can do the same for you. Regular bouts of exercise will fill your body from head to toe with light. Before you take your first step to exercise, your brain will send an impulse of light throughout your body to prepare it to move. In turn, your body will send impulses of light back, causing your brain to send more light throughout your body to increase your respiration and heart rate. In time, your body will be full of light as you exercise dominion over the elements and thus increase your physical capacity to practice self-mastery.

Claim the blessing of this phase—the increased physical capacity to practice self-mastery—by completing what Alma the Younger called a "great check" (Alma 15:17). A "great check" is the act of letting the Lord's light shine upon our personal desires so that we might discover and repent of the "pride of [our] hearts" (Alma 15:17). After completing their own "great check" the people of Sidom chose to divide the light from the darkness of their pride by gathering "together at their sanctuaries to worship God before the altar, watching and praying continually, that they might be delivered from Satan, and from death, and from destruction" (Alma 15:17). Because the people of God during this dispensation were practicing the Law of Moses, their worship at the altar was more than waking up, getting dressed in their Sunday best, and finding a seat in the chapel. Their worship required that they bridle and lead the firstlings of their flocks to the temple to be sacrificed over the refining fire of the altar

Fit for Good

(see Mosiah 2:1–4). This "great check" let the Lord's light into their lives and caused them to physically divide it from the darkness within.

Follow the example of the people of Sidom by checking yourself. Check yourself to ensure that you are letting the Light of Christ into your life physically, in order to increase your physical capacity to practice self-mastery.

Start by circling below how many hours on average you sleep each night. If you don't know, then take the next few days to find out.

Most studies show that adults achieve the full benefits of sleep when they consistently sleep for seven to nine hours a night.[4] In this graph, the white area represents that optimal sleeping time while the dark areas show room for improvement. If your mark is in the dark, decide now to sharpen the division between your days and nights by committing to let the power of the Lord's light protect, renew, and edify your body for seven to nine hours each night.

Now check yourself with this question: Am I wise in what I eat? No matter if you are addicted to food or find very little pleasure in it, when you know why you are eating, your physical capacity to practice self-mastery over what and how much you eat will increase. Keep what can be called a whyse diet by asking and answering, "*Why* am I eating or drinking this?" before each meal or snack.

An honest answer to this question will help you become whyse and therefore enabled to better master *what* and *how much* you eat. For example, as soon as I open the fridge for a late-night snack, the pleasure center in the lower part of my brain will light up and drive me to dive into the last piece of chocolate cake, rather than the fresh grapes next to it because I derive more pleasure from the taste of cake than from grapes.

However, if I stay true to my whyse diet and become whyse to why I want to eat the cake, I will *let* there be light, or in other words, increased neural activity, in the decision-making center in the upper portion of my brain. With this part of my brain activated, I can now *consciously* decide

Divide the Light from the Darkness Within

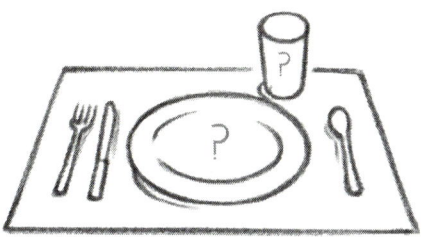

which of these two options will better fill my body with the energy, or "light," of the food which has been "ordained for the constitution, nature, and use of man" (D&C 89:10).

Remember that exercise fills your physical body with impulses of light that enliven every fiber of your being. Regularly filling your body with this light will increase your physical capacity to bridle your natural man's passions. These passions include all of the carnal characteristics of mortality that can roam and run rampant within us, such as depression, vulgarity, anxiety, substance abuse, pornography addiction, arrogance, perfectionism, anger, and fear. Now take a moment to complete a self-check by considering the prominent natural passions that you struggle with. Discretely record your three most prominent natural-man passions in the box titled "Exercise to bridle my" on the upper right side of your Fitness Focus Sphere, but be cautious. When taking stock of your weaknesses and sins, the adversary will try to discourage you. As the master of misery, he will tempt you to focus on all that you are *not* in order to blind you from all that you can *become*.

Defend yourself against his fiery darts by remembering that your personal deficiencies and disobedience do not mark the measure of your creation; however, when bridled, they can become a "beast" (Luke 10:34) on which you carry your broken heart and contrite spirit up the mount of self-mastery to be offered upon the altar of God.

Therefore, I plead with you, increase your physical capacity to bridle your passions by filling your body with the light of regular physical exercise! Remember that a daily dose of physical exercise will fill your body with light—light that can sharpen your resolve to abhor sin, diminish your depression, and alleviate your anxiety.

Fit for Good

```
Exercise to bridle my:
1. _____
2. _____
3. _____
   (Natural man's passions)
```

Measure and report on your efforts to claim the blessing of this phase by marking with a check in your Fitness Focus Sphere each day that you get seven to nine hours of sleep, are whyse in what you eat, and exercise for thirty minutes.

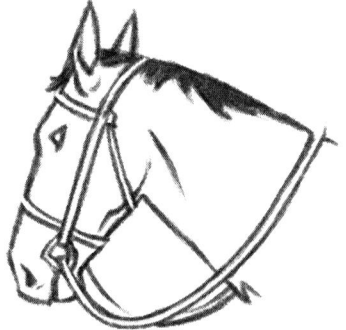

The greater the number of checks in your sphere, the greater your physical capacity to practice the self-mastery necessary to fulfill your fitness focus will be. When you are rested, well fed, and physically active, you will have increased your physical capacity to divide the light from the darkness within.

Consider the example of a young father who chose to claim the blessing of this phase of the Creation. He started his personal self-check by reflecting upon his efforts to physically let the Light of Christ into his life. He realized that each workday he would wake up early, dress himself, go to the kitchen, and start his day by downing a caffeine-loaded can

Divide the Light from the Darkness Within

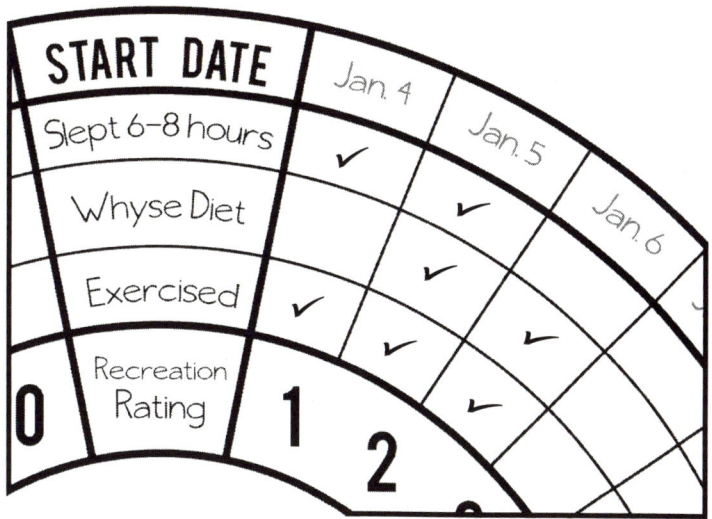

of soda. He would then eat breakfast and head to work. After work, he would come home, eat dinner with his family, help put the children to bed, and then "recover" from his long day by spending some time on the TV, computer, or his smart phone. He started his whyse diet and asked himself—*Why do I down a can of this soda every morning?* He realized that his morning sustenance was really a morning substance that he had become dependent upon to keep himself alert and awake throughout his workday.

He downed the soda each morning for the caffeine that covered the physical consequence of his late and idle nights—the late and idle nights that served as the reserve on which his dominate natural man's passions found room to run. He decided to claim the blessing of this phase by measuring and reporting on his efforts to physically illuminate his life with the Light of Christ. He traded in his late nights for seven hours of divine sleep. He conquered his caffeine habit with a whyse diet and an early morning bout of exercise to better bridle his natural man's passions. His daily focus became single to the glory of God and filled his body "full of light" (Luke 11:34–36), increasing his physical capacity to practice self-mastery.

Fit for Good

You can do the same. Let the Master's light physically illuminate your life and increase your physical capacity to practice the self-mastery that will chase the darkness of the natural man from within you (see D&C 50:25). As you measure and report on your efforts to enter His rest each night, remain whyse to what you eat, and fill your body with the light of regular exercise, you will be ready to claim the blessing of the third phase of the Creation. The third phase will *beautify* your exercise efforts and increase your physical capacity to fill the measure of your creation with the fulness of joy found only in the fourth phase.

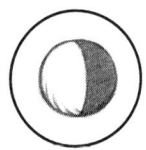

Divide the light from the darkness within by entering into the Lord's rest, eating whysely, and bridling your passions with exercise to *increase your physical capacity to practice self-mastery*.

… Fit for Good

LINE UPON LINE SUMMARY

On Your Mark

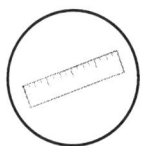

Receive God's image. Remember, your body is *the measure of your creation*—the physical manifestation of your potential to become like God.

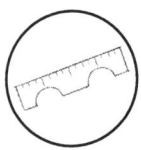

Yoke yourself to Christ when you exercise. Remember, *His yoke will enable* the measure of your creation to be filled with a fulness of joy.

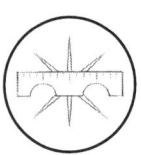

Invite the Spirit to be with you when you exercise. Remember, *His power will quicken* the measure of your creation so you can experience a fulness of joy.

Divide the Light from the Darkness Within

LINE UPON LINE SUMMARY

Get Set

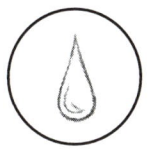
Sweat in the wilderness of regular exercise. The *sweat of your brow* is the manifestation of your effort to subject the fallen elements of your body to your divine spirit.

Defend against the adversary's fiery darts. *Watch and pray* for protection against the darts of physical lust, latency, and limits that will fill the measure of your creation with misery.

Experiment upon the word of God. By *exercising faith in the word of God*, you can increase your physical capacity to fill the measure of your creation with a fulness of joy.

LINE UPON LINE SUMMARY

Go!

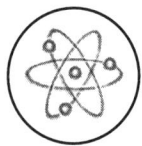

Create a *fitness focus statement*. Select a *fitness fellow* to return and report to about your efforts to claim the blessings of exercising according to the Lord's pattern of creation.

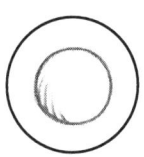

Form your flesh by exercising to *increase your physical capacity to act*.

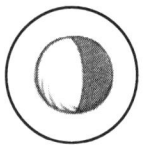

Divide the light from the darkness within by entering into the Lord's rest, eating whysely, and bridling your passions with exercise to *increase your physical capacity to practice self-mastery*.

CHAPTER 10

Beautify Your Fitness

Six o'clock in the morning and about 95 degrees—that was the time and scorching temperature for our weekly Saturday morning three-on-three basketball game in Tempe, Arizona. On this particular morning, my father, brother-in-law Jared, and cousin Steve came with me to the old courts in our neighborhood park. We all chuckled when my good friend Ryan, showed up with two of his cousins, Spencer and Preston. My father graciously offered to sit out the first few games so we could hold a best-of-three Rapier versus Tenney tournament. I sized up our competition and began to feel quite confident that together my vertically blessed brother-in-law and sharp-shooting cousin would cut and serve the Rapiers a nice piece of humble pie.

In game one, we found early success by giving the ball to Jared who used his tall, strong, Idaho-farm-boy frame to score several quick points. The Rapiers quickly adjusted and double-teamed Jared. This left Steve open, and he used his smooth stroke to drain several threes. I could smell the humble pie a-cookin'. Series score: 1–0, Tenneys ahead.

Game two became a circus. The Rapiers were the performers, and we were their props. Channeling the Harlem Globetrotters, they dribbled, passed, drove, and scored with ease. I glanced over at my dad. I was surprised to see him on his feet applauding their amazing play. Hold the humble pie. Series score: 1–1, tied up.

With the series tied, game three carried all the weight. Each team huddled together to talk strategy. Because they won the last game, the Rapiers started with the ball, and with a few perfect passes and moves, Ryan was open for an uncontested three. Game score: 3–0, Rapiers. Jared passed the ball in to Steve, who drove hard to the basket. Preston collapsed to help and left a trailing Jared open for an easy layup. Game score: 3–2, Rapiers. Determined to contribute to the game, I stepped up my defense, stole the ball from Spencer, and quickly passed it to a wide-open Steve on the wing for a three. Game score: 5–3, Tenneys.

As the final game went on, each team took turns leading the game. Amazing plays by both teams increased the tension of our basketball battle in the now one-hundred-degree heat. Then I saw and felt something different. The tension of the game gave way. Not because of an injury, but because our purpose for playing shifted from trying to glorify our team by winning the game to enjoying the glory of the game itself. Our capacity to play better basketball seemed to increase as we cheered each other along with shouts, such as, "Sweet shot!" and "Nice block." I thought to myself, *Now I know what a game of basketball will be like in heaven.* Our game to twenty-one points went way beyond twenty-one points because each team served the other with their best play until the game was brought to a close by a contested three-pointer that slipped perfectly through the metal net. That shot sealed in my mind not a final score, but a forever memory of the most *beautiful* game I have ever played.

BEAUTIFY

After forming the earth and dividing the light from the darkness upon it, the Lord then began the third phase of the Creation by *beautifying* the earth. First, He gathered the waters together and caused the "dry land" to appear (Moses 2:9). This gathering and moving of the great waters created the beautiful and various landscapes of mountains, valleys, and flowing streams that we enjoy throughout the earth. After he gathered the water and dry land, the Lord then created and placed every form of life on the earth (see Moses 2:24). The combination of His unique and diverse creations gave variety to the earth and made it beautiful.

Why did the Lord beautify the earth? Why didn't he just create the earth to be a bland collection of dirt, water, cacti, and brussels sprouts? In section 59 of the Doctrine and Covenants, we learn the answer.

> Yea, and the herb, and the *good things* which come of the earth, whether for food or for raiment, or for houses, or for barns, or for orchards, or for gardens, or for vineyards; Yea, *all things which come of the earth*, in the season thereof, *are* made for the benefit and the use of man, *both to please the eye and to gladden the heart*; Yea, for food and for raiment, for taste and for smell, *to strengthen the body and to enliven the soul.* (D&C 59:17–19; emphasis added)

God *beautified* the earth, with all its varied mountains, valleys, and vegetation, not just to sustain life but to please the eye, gladden the heart, strengthen the body, and enliven the soul. In other words, He beautified the earth so that we might find joy in its beauty.

We participate in the third phase of the Creation by *beautifying* our efforts to exercise dominion over the elements of our bodies. The word "beautify" means to make something physically more pleasurable or satisfying. Many of the most popular fitness trends today have found great success in this phase by providing individuals opportunities to beautify their exercise efforts. This has been done by incorporating Latin dance, extreme relays, extreme obstacles, and splashes of color into our efforts to get fit. The joy meted in this phase is greater than the joy meted in the previous phases because of the endless ways we can beautify our fitness efforts. However, over time, the joy experienced in this phase will become *linearly limited* if we beautify our exercise efforts to *give* joy only to *ourselves*.

Fit for Good

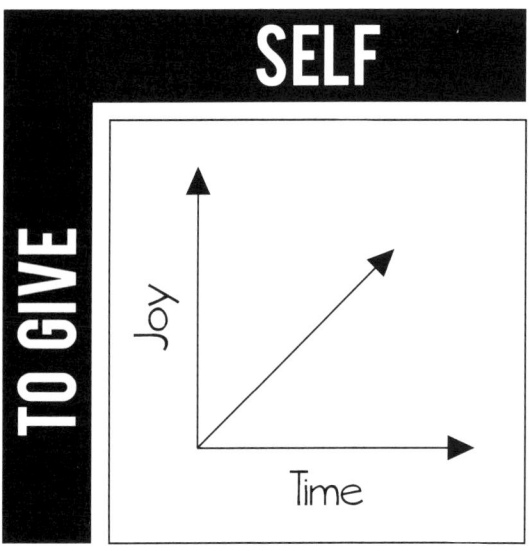

Consider the parable of the talents that Christ gave to His disciples: "For the kingdom of heaven is as a man traveling into a far country, who called his own servants, and delivered unto them his goods. And unto one he gave five talents, to another two, and to another one; to every man according to his several ability; and straightway took his journey" (Matthew 25:14–15).

Like the servants in the parable, we too have been given "the goods" of God—our specific talents which are expressions of the divine DNA within each of us. The adversary knows these divine talents can give us joy and will send his fiery darts to either suppress or swindle "the goods" that God has given you to beautify your fitness efforts. In this parable, the adversary's fiery darts hit their mark within the heart of the last servant. When the Master returned and asked for an accounting of what the servant did with the master's goods, the servant replied, "I was *afraid*, and went and *hid* thy talent in the earth" (Matthew 25:25; emphasis added). When it comes to our efforts to claim the blessing of this phase, the adversary will tempt us to bury the talents that the Father has given us under the fear and fallacy that we don't have the time or energy to beautify our fitness efforts. These exercise excuses are the fill by which we bury—and thus suppress—the God-given talents that can enable us to beautify our exercise efforts (see D&C 60:13).

If the adversary is unsuccessful at tempting us to suppress our talents, he will then try to swindle them from us. This happens when we beautify our fitness efforts "just for fun." Keep in mind that exercising for fun is not bad in and of itself. I am confident the Lord found great personal joy as He exercised dominion over the elements to beautify the earth; however, this was not His primary purpose for doing so. We know His primary purpose in beautifying the earth was "for the benefit and the use of man, both to please the eye and to gladden the heart . . . to strengthen the body and to enliven the soul[s]" of His children (D&C 59:18–19). We too can find great personal joy when we beautify our exercise efforts. However, when our participation in a Latin dance program, extreme relay race, obstacle course, or glow-in-the-dark run is done "just for fun" and for only "Number One," our joy will be linearly limited because that joy can lead us to becoming forever "wanton" for more fun (James 5:5).

You can defend against the adversary's attacks by focusing your efforts on claiming the blessing of this phase that will increase your physical capacity to fulfill your fitness focus rather than focusing on the *linearly limited* joy found in this phase.

GO!

Let's return to the parable of the talents and learn how to claim the blessing of this phase by following the examples of the first two servants. We learn that each servant was first given a number of talents "according to his several ability" (Matthew 25:15). The Master gave the first servant five talents; the second, two; and the last, one. The first servant "went and traded with the same, and made them other five talents. And likewise he that had received two, he also gained other two" (Matthew 25:16–17). These two servants did not bury their talents; they *traded* them to literally "*re-create*" them—to create five more for the first and two more for the second.

Fit for Good

The Master returned and individually blessed both servants, saying, "Well done, thou good and faithful servant: thou hast been faithful over a few things, I will make thee ruler over many things: enter thou into the joy of thy lord" (Matthew 25:21). They were blessed with an increase in their stewardship, an increase that would enable them to do more good and thus enter into the joy of the Lord. When you exercise to re-create the talents God has given you, you will be blessed with an increase as well—an *increase in your physical capacity to do good.*

Recreational exercise can increase your physical capacity to do more good because it can serve as a "safety [valve] to keep the tension down and the spirit up," and increase your "capacity to reason, to act, and to find purpose in life."[1] Recreational exercise through "music, literature, art, dance, drama, athletics—all can provide entertainment to enrich one's life and *further* consecrate it."[2] The capacity to "further consecrate" is the blessing of this phase that will help you fulfill your fitness focus.

I had the opportunity to increase my capacity to "further consecrate" on an early Saturday morning when my brother Tom unexpectedly invited me to tackle Whiskey Row once again. This time it wasn't to run down it in a pair of old cowboy boots, but rather to jog along it in the annual Whiskey Row 10k race. I was genuinely excited about the invitation, even though I knew the race was going to be difficult for my short and stocky sprinter's body. I was excited because for more than six miles I was going to have the opportunity to re-create my talent to mingle with and make new friends as my brother and I pounded the pavement with the other runners. After sharing our plan with our selfless wives, we laced up our running shoes, drove down to Whiskey Row, and registered for the race. We pinned our race numbers on and began to warm up. That warm up didn't last long, however, because we noticed family members and friends at the race as well. My face beamed from ear to ear as I began to re-create my talent as I embraced extended family members and friends from long ago.

Though our hearts were warmed up when the race started, our bodies were not. Therefore, Tom and I used the first few hundred yards to ease into the race. The pace was perfect for my stocky little frame; however, I could see that Tom was holding back his slender and swift body to remain with me.

"Enjoy the race at your pace," I suggested.

"See you at the finish line," he said, shifting into a gear that I could only dream about.

After a few hundred yards of running, my bowling ball of a body began to roll slower and slower down the road. My pitiful pace caused me to notice the grunts, groans, and deep breaths of those around me who were struggling through the wilderness experience of their run.

Then the Spirit invited me to look once again. I began to see the *beauty* of the moment. I was witnessing hundreds of God's children exercising together, subjecting the fallen elements of their bodies to their divine spirits. At that moment, I had a deep desire to make it more beautiful. So I took the talent to mingle that God gave me and began to "trade" it with those around me. I started by encouraging the eighty-year-old veteran who flashed a smile as he passed by me in his army boots and fatigues. Though my body was burdened, my spirit was lifted as I cheered on the few I passed and the many who passed me. I was grateful for the sweat beading down my face because it provided cover for my tears of joy. Quickened by the Spirit, I sped up my pace and looked forward to the finish line knowing that my brother was waiting there for me.

It is important to re-create your talents as you exercise "according to [your] several [personal exercise] abilities" (Matthew 25:15). These abilities are what make up our exercise preferences. Many of us view regular physical exercise as a "hard man" (Matthew 25:24) that requires us to push aside our fitness preferences as we struggle through the pressure, panting, and pain of exercise activity that we don't particularly enjoy. Many of us may even falter under the pressure and pain. This "hard man" perspective, if not overcome, can only provide us with a pile of fitness failures to bury our talents beneath.

Limit the pileup and prepare to re-create your talents by discovering your current exercise preferences. There are three primary exercise preferences that will significantly influence your ability to re-create your talents as you exercise. They are our exercise *sociality, setting,* and *strategy* preferences. The primary sociality preference constitutes our desire to exercise alone or with others. The primary setting preference deals with your desire to exercise in a staged or a spontaneous environment. The primary strategy preference deals with you desire to compete or collaborate as you exercise.

Discover your primary exercise preferences by circling the word that describes best your exercise preference on each side of the three continuums below.

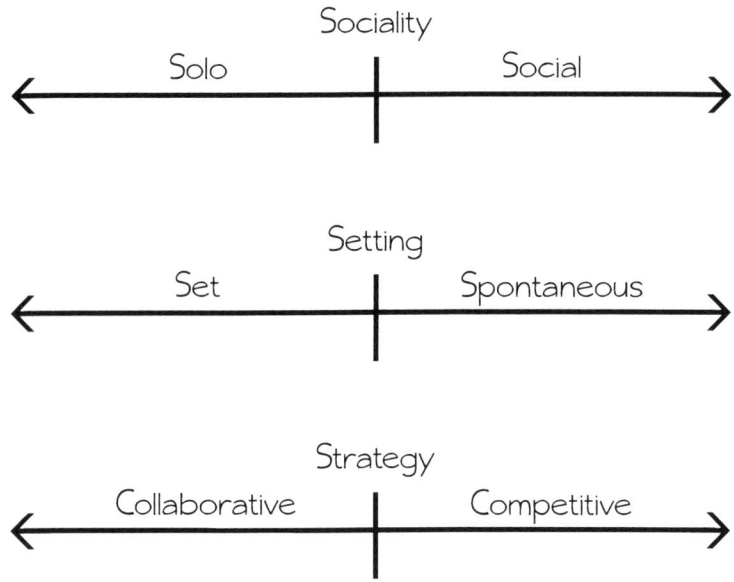

Record your current primary exercise performances in the boxes below.

Sociality	Setting	Strategy

Once you have determined your primary exercise preferences, you can find some exercise suggestions below.

Solo, Set, and Collaborative
With these exercise preferences, you will likely enjoy exercise activities that are done alone, that are plain, simple, and proven, and that are for a personal goal. Exercise activities that you might prefer include running, walking, cycling, yoga, and swimming.

Solo, Spontaneous, and Collaborative
With these exercise preferences, you will likely enjoy exercise activities that limit interaction with others, that are well-established activities but still keep you guessing, and that help you reach your personal exercise goals. Exercise activities that you might prefer include trail running, mountain biking, hiking, interval training, and Pilates.

Solo, Set, and Competitive
With these exercise preferences, you will likely enjoy private exercise activities that pit yourself against a previously set personal record, such as a previous bench press weight or mile run time. Exercises that you might prefer include cardio workouts, weight lifting, running, cycling, and swimming.

Solo, Spontaneous, and Competitive
With these exercise preferences, you will likely enjoy personal exercise activities that place you in a position to conquer a variety of physical obstacles, like the stairs at work, a nearby mountain peak, or the monstrous hill on the way home. Exercise activities that you might prefer include trail running, cycling, hiking, rock climbing, and mountain biking.

Social, Set, and Collaborative
With these exercise preferences, you will likely enjoy joining with friends or fitness instructors who will help you engage in simple and proven exercise activities that will help you reach your fitness goals. Exercise activities that you might prefer include strength and cardio training at the gym, walking groups, and running clubs.

Social, Spontaneous, and Collaborative
With these exercise preferences, you will likely enjoy exercise activities that place you in a position to meet new people and participate in a variety of exercise activities. Exercise activities that you might prefer include joining a hiking club, a boot camp, a color run, or a studio with varied exercise classes, such as tai chi, yoga, Pilates, and dance.

Social, Set, and Competitive
With these exercise preferences, you will likely enjoy personal exercise activities that place you in a position to compete with others in simple and structured settings. Exercise activities that you might prefer include martial arts, racquet sports, training groups, relay races, cycling races, and strength training competitions.

Social, Spontaneous, and Competitive
With these exercise preferences, you will likely enjoy personal exercise activities that place you in a position to compete with others in varied settings. Exercise activities that you might prefer include team sports, such as basketball or soccer; obstacle course competitions; triathlons; trail running; and mountain bike races.

Beautify Your Fitness

Now remember these are your *current* exercise preferences; they may change over time. However, by knowing your preferences you can confidently participate in those activities that will help you enjoy recreating your talents and thus claim the blessing of this phase.

Prepare to claim this blessing by listing below the talents with which God has blessed you. I recognize that this might be difficult for some to do, so ask for help from your fitness fellow, family members, and close friends. Ask them to share with you the talents they believe the Lord has given to you. If you have received a patriarchal blessing, read it and look for the talents that God has given to you.

_____
_____
_____
_____
_____
_____
_____
_____
_____
_____
_____
_____
_____
_____
_____

Fit for Good

Now with your fitness fellow's help, select three talents that you could re-create according to your exercise preferences and record them in the box titled "Exercise to re-create my" on your Fitness Focus Sphere.

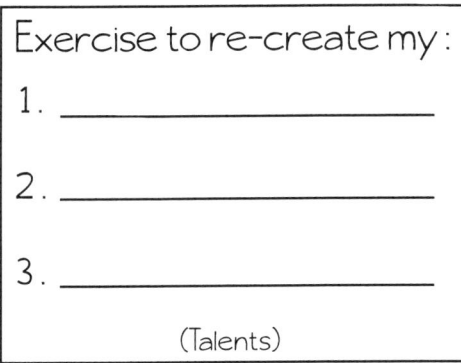

For example, if you have a solo, set, and collaborative exercise preference and have a talent for dance, rather than signing up for an uncomfortable class at the studio, find a dance DVD you can exercise with at home.

If you have a solo, set, and competitive exercise preference and you have a talent for math, then figure out a way to record the number of miles you move, calories you burn, and steps you take so you can set several personal records that you can work to best during the next day, week, or month.

If you have a solo, spontaneous, and competitive exercise preference and an artistic talent, then look for the beauty of God's art as you conquer the mountain range in your area.

If you have a solo, spontaneous, and collaborative exercise preference and talent for music, then listen to the works of various music masters as you jog different trails or parks in your area.

If you have a social, set, and collaborative exercise preference and you have been given the talent to comfort others, then invite a friend in need to join you on your daily walks.

If you have a social, set, and competitive exercise preference and a talent for organization, then organize a group to train for a local competitive run.

Beautify Your Fitness

If you have a social, spontaneous, and collaborative exercise preference and a talent for cooking, then learn how to cook a post-training meal for your fellow boot camp members.

If you have a social, spontaneous, and competitive exercise preference and a talent for teaching, then coach your child's soccer team and join them in the drills you have them do.

If your talents seem to have nothing to do with exercise, remember that you are a child of the "most creative Being in the universe."[3] You have the ability to re-create with the talents God has blessed you with!

Now claim the blessing of this phase by *returning* and *reporting* on your efforts to beautify your exercise. After exercising to re-create a talent for two weeks, rate the likelihood that you would exercise to re-create that talent for two *more* weeks on a scale of one to ten—the greater the number, the greater your desire. Record that number on your Fitness Focus Sphere.

The beauty of this simple scale is that no matter what your score is, you can use it to better beautify your fitness efforts with a little *whyse* discernment. If your score is greater than seven, great! Share with your fitness fellow *why* the re-creation of this talent excites you to exercise and try to magnify it. For example, if you enjoyed hiking to re-create your talent for art, then make a plan to magnify it by joining a hiking club.

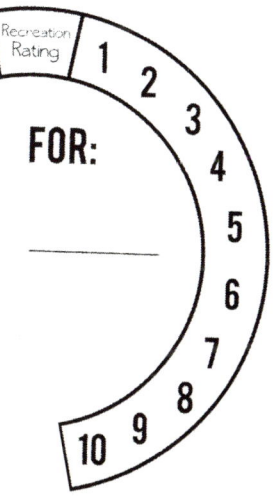

If your score is less than four, again share with your fitness fellow *why* and try to eliminate the factors that caused your score to be so low. For example, if joining your friend at the gym to re-create your talent for socialization did little to excite you to exercise because of the overwhelming competitive and physique focus found there, then reconsider your current exercise preference and invite your friend to join you at the local park for a workout. If that doesn't work, then pick another talent and try again.

If your score is somewhere in the middle of four and seven, share with your fitness fellow *why* your score wasn't *lower*. Take your answer and magnify it. For example, if listening to conference talks while running on the treadmill to re-create your love for the word of God had a lower rating, but there was a certain topic or speaker that made a difference in your run, then create a playlist of that speaker or that topic and give it a try again.

Now remember, the joy that comes from beautifying your fitness efforts by recreating your talents can go a long way in fueling your efforts to get physically fit. However, this joy is linearly limited. It is the blessing of this phase combined with the previous two that will enable you to fulfill your fitness focus and prepare you to participate in the fourth and final phase of the Creation, the phase that will *multiply* your fitness efforts and fill the measure of your creation with a fulness of joy.

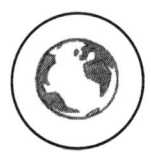

Beautify your fitness efforts by recreating your talents as you exercise to *increase your capacity to do good*.

LINE UPON LINE SUMMARY

On Your Mark

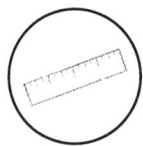

Receive God's image. Remember, your body is *the measure of your creation*—the physical manifestation of your potential to become like God.

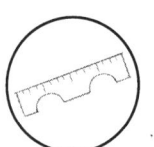

Yoke yourself to Christ when you exercise. Remember, *His yoke will enable* the measure of your creation to be filled with a fulness of joy.

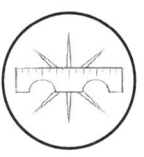

Invite the Spirit to be with you when you exercise. Remember, *His power will quicken* the measure of your creation so you can experience a fulness of joy.

LINE UPON LINE SUMMARY

Get Set

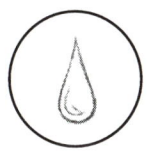

Sweat in the wilderness of regular exercise. The *sweat of your brow* is the manifestation of your effort to subject the fallen elements of your body to your divine spirit.

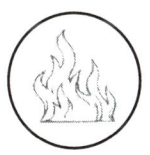

Defend against the adversary's fiery darts. *Watch and pray* for protection against the darts of physical lust, latency, and limits that will fill the measure of your creation with misery.

Experiment upon the word of God. By *exercising faith in the word of God*, you can increase your physical capacity to fill the measure of your creation with a fulness of joy.

LINE UPON LINE SUMMARY

Go!

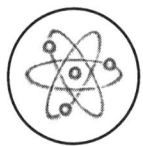

Create a *fitness focus statement*. Select a *fitness fellow* to return and report to about your efforts to claim the blessings of exercising according to the Lord's pattern of creation.

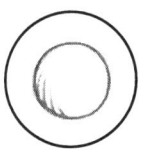

Form your flesh by exercising to *increase your physical capacity to act*.

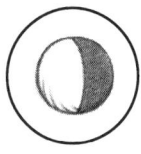

Divide the light from the darkness within by entering into the Lord's rest, eating whysely, and bridling your passions with exercise to *increase your physical capacity to practice self-mastery*.

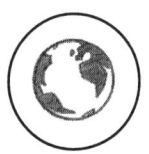

Beautify your fitness efforts by recreating your talents as you exercise to *increase your capacity to do good*.

CHAPTER 11

Multiply the Blessings

I could hear them whisper my name. They were coming for me. I sat up and said a quick prayer as my freshman body coiled in fear. Earlier that week, I had accepted my varsity track coach's invitation to travel with the team and compete in the regional championships—in the shot put, an unlikely event for a short and scrawny boy. However, God blessed me with the quickness to spin fast enough to throw the twelve-pound metal ball a decent distance.

Now I wished I hadn't come. Our coach had sent us into the home team's locker room to escape the scorching heat of Phoenix, Arizona. Once in the locker room, I separated myself from the others to catch up on my homework. All went well for a while, but then I heard it, my teammates whispering my name. "I bet Tenney has never seen anything like this."

My heart began to race. I crept around the bay where I was working to see what was going on. I recoiled quickly. One of my teammates had brought a mini TV and video player combo and a pornographic video. I knew I had to flee, but the TV and its captives were parked in the middle of the locker room blocking my escape. I instead gathered my stuff and slipped to the far end of the locker room. I hunkered down and tried to distract myself with my homework.

I heard my teammates whisper my name again.

Two of the largest boys on our team peaked around the corner of my bay. "Hey Tenney, we want to show you something," they said.

I mustered the courage to say, "I'm not interested, guys." They came toward me, not willing to take no for an answer. I stood up and did my best Nephi impersonation, commanding them to "touch me not" (1 Nephi 17:48). Lacking the faith to stretch forth my hand and shock them, I sat back down and held firm to the locker bench. They chuckled, grabbed my feet, and tried to peel me away from the bench. In desperation, I called out for help. The Lord provided rescue.

"Hey, what's going on?" asked Stan Gologoski, our track team captain. Startled, my enemies quickly let my legs go.

"Nothing," they replied as they cowered in the shadow of his six-foot-three, two-hundred-plus-pound frame. "Leave Tenney alone, and get rid of the TV," he commanded. The boys obeyed. I could feel the powers of hell shake in his Captain Moroni-like presence. Stan approached me to make sure I was all right. I thanked him and did my best to hold back my tears of joy.

MULTIPLY

Let's return to the mount with Moses. Moses was blessed to see the fulness of this final phase of the Creation: the multiply phase—the phase that filled the measure of the earth's creation.

> Moses cast his eyes and beheld the earth, yea, even all of it; and there was not a particle of it which he did not behold, discerning it by the Spirit of God. And he beheld also the inhabitants thereof, and there was not a soul which he beheld not; and he discerned them by the Spirit of God; and their numbers were great, even numberless as the sand upon the sea shore. (Moses 1:27–28)

These numberless souls are the fruit of the final phase of the Creation, the phase in which the earth was *multiplied* "to bring to pass the immortality and eternal life of man" (Moses 1:39).

Adam and Eve ushered in this final phase of the Creation when they chose to join the Lord in His labors. They partook of the forbidden

Multiply the Blessings

fruit so they could "*multiply*" (Moses 2:28; emphasis added) that "men might be" (2 Nephi 2:25). From that time forward, Adam and Eve and all mankind began to form, divide, and beautify the fallen earth "by the sweat of [their imperfect brows]" in order to *multiply* the blessings of their posterity (Moses 5:1–2).

In the meridian of time, the Savior came, and by the sweat of His perfect brow He *multiplied* the blessings of all mankind through His infinite sacrifice in the garden and upon the cross.

This final phase is founded upon the *multiplying* effects of selfless sacrifice. Adam and Eve sacrificed their immortality and presence with our Father so that man might be. The Savior sacrificed His immortality and presence with His Father so that all men might live again with God.

You can do the same; you can multiply your fitness efforts by exercising dominion over the elements of your body *to give* of yourself to bless the lives of *others*. The joy from this final phase is an *exponential* joy, as depicted in the graph below. It is the eternal joy that our Father in Heaven experiences. This joy is not found in His omnipotent capacity to *form*, *divide* and *beautify* "all things" (D&C 38:1–3), but in His eternal efforts to give of Himself "to bring to pass the immortality and eternal

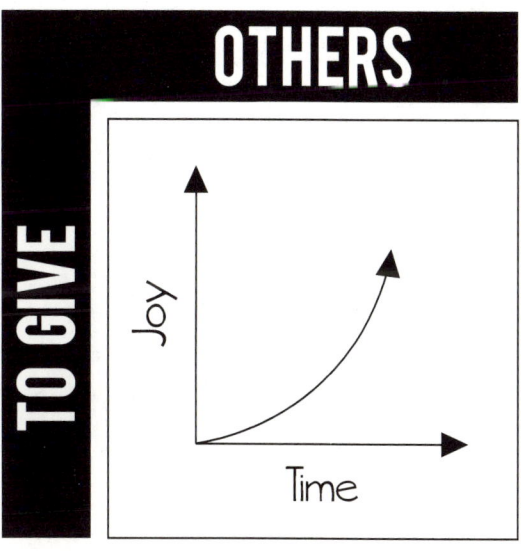

life" of His children (Moses 1:39). You can experience this eternal joy in your fitness efforts by exercising to give of yourself to bless the lives of others.

The adversary knows this, but here is the good news: there is *nothing* he can do to tempt you in this phase. If you remain true to your fitness focus in each phase, you will increase your physical capacity to act, practice self-mastery, and do good so that you can bless the lives of others. When your fitness efforts are focused on blessing the lives of others, you will be yoked to Christ when you exercise, and because you are yoked to Christ, the adversary's fiery darts will be powerless against you (see 1 Nephi 22:26 and Helaman 5:12). That is why, unlike the other phases, the eternal joy found in this phase is also the blessing that we must seek.

The efforts of the four good men who physically bore the burden of their paralytic brother as recorded in Mark chapter 2 are great examples to us of how to physically participate in this phase of the Creation. At least one of these four men undoubtedly had heard of the miraculous healings performed by Christ in Capernaum and returned to share the good news of this great healer with his paralytic brother. Oh what joy must have filled their hearts to know that he could be made whole.

Each man secured a corner of the paralytic's bed and carried him to Christ. Upon arrival at the home where Christ was teaching, they found it impossible to enter, due to the throng of people that had come to see Christ. The situation did not deter them, and these men continued to exercise their faith by physically lifting their bother up onto the roof of the house. They then "uncovered the roof where [Christ] was: and when they had broken it up, they let down the bed wherein the sick of the palsy lay" (Mark 2:4). What joy must the Savior have felt as he witnessed the physical efforts of these four men in behalf of their brother? His joy must have been full as the men exemplified unto all in the house—and to all that would ever read this passage of scripture—how to *physically* take upon ourselves the yoke of Christ.

Multiply the Blessings

"Here am I, send me" (Abraham 3:27)	*Like Christ, these men volunteered*
"Surely he has borne our griefs, and carried our sorrows" (Mosiah 4:4)	*to physically bear the burden of their brother*
"I am the way, the truth, and the life: no man cometh unto the Father, but by me" (John 14:6)	*so that he might have a way to come unto God.*
"And my Father sent me that I might be lifted up upon the cross; and after that I had been lifted up upon the cross, that I might draw all men unto me, that as I have been lifted up by men even so should men be lifted up by the Father" (3 Nephi 27:14)	*They physically lifted themselves up so they could lift their brother up to be closer to God.*
"And thus God breaketh the bands of death, having gained the victory over death; giving the Son power to make intercession for the children of men" (Mosiah 15:8)	*They broke through the barrier of the rooftop that physically separated their brother from the presence of God.*

These four men multiplied their fitness efforts and became "true yokefellow[s]" (Philippians 4:3) with Christ by exercising dominion over the elements of their bodies to help bear their brother's burden. You can choose to multiply your fitness efforts by magnifying your fitness focus. You can do this by exercising not to "save" your life, but to "lose" it as you exercise to bless the life of a specific individual or individuals (Luke 17:33). By doing so, you will claim the blessing of this phase—*the increased physical capacity to experience a fulness of joy.*

GO!

As a young child, I remember my father sharing with me the following story about a man who participated in this phase of the Creation. It touched me then and still inspires me today.

Fit for Good

During a heavy snowstorm on January 13, 1982, Air Florida Flight 90 crashed into the 14th Street Bridge and plummeted into the icy, frigid Potomac River shortly after takeoff. The crash took the lives of seventy of its passengers, four of its crew, and four motorists on the bridge. Six of the passengers miraculously survived the initial crash and hoped for rescue in the ice-choked Potomac by working their way to the tail section of the plane, which was above the surface of the water. Their answer came in the form of a rescue helicopter that lowered a line to the survivors. The first survivor to grab the line was quickly dragged to safety. The helicopter returned and then dropped the line into the hands of Arland D. Williams. For a brief moment, he held in his hands his future, his chance to see his family again, to "save" his life, yet he chose to pass the line to flight attendant Kelly Duncan who was then safely dragged to shore.

The helicopter returned and then lowered Arland two lifelines to his future. He again passed them on. He gave the first line to Joe Stiley, who was holding tight to a trembling Priscilla Tirado. He gave the second line to Nikki Felch, Stiley's coworker. With Stiley and Felch holding tight, the helicopter began to drag the trio through the body-beating blocks of ice toward the waiting arms of those on shore. The beatings and fatigue were too much for Tirado and Felch, who fell back into the water. Lenny Skutnik, a brave bystander, stripped off his outer layer of clothes and dove in and successfully rescued Tirado. The helicopter then returned to where Felch had fallen. Paramedic Gene Windsor stepped out onto the skid of the helicopter, grabbed Felch, and slumped her over the helicopter's skid. After saving Felch, the helicopter returned for Williams. The tailpiece of the plane had rolled. Williams was gone.[1]

Roger Rosenblatt wrote,

> So the man in the water [Arland] had his own natural powers. He could not make ice storms, or freeze the water until it froze the blood. But he could hand life over to a stranger, and that is a power of nature too. The man in the water pitted himself against an implacable, impersonal enemy; he fought it with charity; and he held it to a standoff. He was the best we can do.[2]

Multiply the Blessings

Williams's heroic act in the icy Potomac is a powerful example of how to participate in and claim the blessing of the final phase of the Creation. He multiplied his physical efforts by choosing to bear the burden of death for another. In that frigid water, Williams fully subjected the elements of his fallen body to his divine spirit. With each pass of the lifeline, he yoked his water-soaked body to Christ, increasing his *capacity to experience a fulness of joy*. Undoubtedly, he felt that fulness of joy when he was "taken home" to the loving arms of the "God who gave [him] life" (Alma 40:11).

You don't have to plunge into the icy waters of the Potomac to participate in this final phase of the Creation. You can multiply your fitness efforts by exercising to bless a person in need.

Consider a married couple where the husband struggles with an addiction to pornography. Together, they decide to help bear one another's burden by setting a goal to hike out of their "valley of sorrow" *together* (2 Nephi 4:26). They make a plan to pray, ponder, and discuss their relationship together as they physically prepare in six weeks to complete a rim-to-rim hike through the Grand Canyon. They train together to increase his physical capacity to practice self-mastery in hopes that when they climb out of the canyon, a portion, if not all, of his weapon of war (pornography) will remain buried at the bottom of the Great Creator's Canyon (see Alma 24:19).

For example, I know of a father who exercised to help bear the burden of his daughter suffering from obsessive-compulsive disorder. At home, when her obsession surfaced, he would go on a light jog with her to help her chase away the darkness of obsessive thoughts by filling her body with the light of exercise. These runs yoked the both of them to Christ as they pulled together to ease her burden.

Consider the busy mother that realizes that her young son, a middle child, is in need of her attention. She decides to multiply her fitness efforts by playing soccer, jumping on the trampoline, and chasing lizards with him throughout the week. Consider the father who rides his bike to work to save gas money so he can pay for his daughter to attend dance class. Consider the group of extended family members that decide to lose weight together, not with a purpose of seeing who can lose the most, but with a purpose of setting a goal to "hand down" the collective pounds they lose in the form of food to the local food bank. Consider the individual, family, or community that chooses to participate in one of the many walk, run, and ride-a-thons in behalf of those who carry the burden of a certain illness or condition.

Take a moment to magnify your fitness focus by listing below the names of those you love and the burdens they are carrying.

Name	Burdens
_____	_____
_____	_____
_____	_____
_____	_____

Now prayerfully consider ways that you might multiply your fitness efforts to help bear the burden of one of the individuals above. Again, remember you are a child of the Great Creator, so be creative! If you find this difficult, counsel with your fitness fellow for ideas. Place the name of the individual you selected in the center of your Fitness Focus Sphere.

Share with your fitness fellow your plan to multiply your fitness efforts by exercising to bless the life of this individual for the next four weeks. If you complete your efforts for this individual before the four weeks is up, multiply your efforts and select another to serve. At the end of your four-week cycle, return and report by sharing with your fitness fellow how your efforts increased your capacity to experience a fulness of joy. It is that simple. When you multiply your fitness efforts by exercising to bless the life of another, you will increase your physical capacity to experience the exponential and eternal joy of this phase (see D&C 109:76). It is the joy that was experienced by the four who physically bore their brother's burden and brought him to the feet of the Savior. It is the joy that was

Multiply the Blessings

experienced by Arland D. Williams who physically bore the burden of death in behalf of his brother and sisters in the icy waters of the Potomac. It is the joy that was experienced by a strong Moroni-like track captain who bore the burden of fear for a scrawny freshman; the joy experienced by the two who bore the burden of their Fall so that you and I might be; and it was the joy experienced by the One who has born the burdens of us all so that we might have the opportunity to become physically *fit for good*.

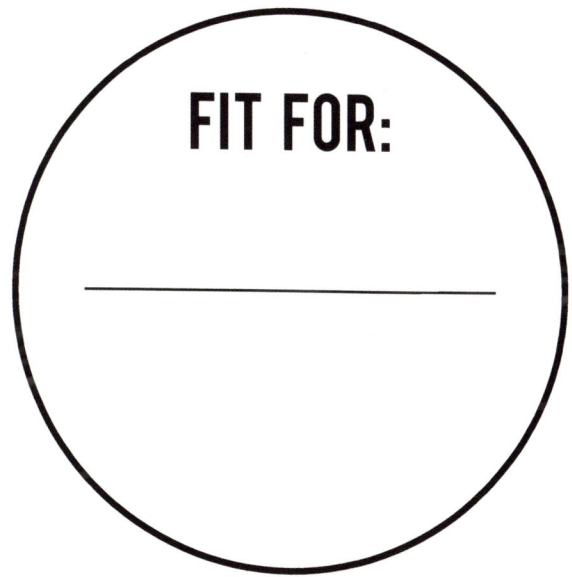

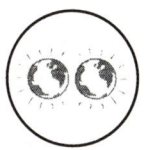 Multiply your fitness efforts by exercising to bless the life of another to *increase your physical capacity to experience a fulness of joy.*

LINE UPON LINE SUMMARY

On Your Mark

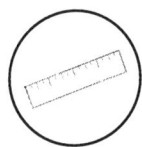

Receive God's image. Remember, your body is *the measure of your creation*—the physical manifestation of your potential to become like God.

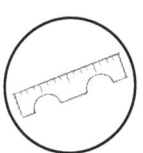

Yoke yourself to Christ when you exercise. Remember, *His yoke will enable* the measure of your creation to be filled with a fulness of joy.

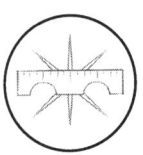

Invite the Spirit to be with you when you exercise. Remember, *His power will quicken* the measure of your creation so you can experience a fulness of joy.

Multiply the Blessings

LINE UPON LINE SUMMARY

Get Set

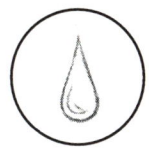
Sweat in the wilderness of regular exercise. The *sweat of your brow* is the manifestation of your effort to subject the fallen elements of your body to your divine spirit.

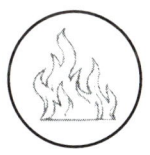
Defend against the adversary's fiery darts. *Watch and pray* for protection against the darts of physical lust, latency, and limits that will fill the measure of your creation with misery.

Experiment upon the word of God. By *exercising faith in the word of God*, you can increase your physical capacity to fill the measure of your creation with a fulness of joy.

Fit for Good

LINE UPON LINE SUMMARY

Go!

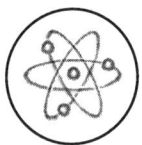

Create a *fitness focus statement*. Select a *fitness fellow* to return and report to about your efforts to claim the blessings of exercising according to the Lord's pattern of creation.

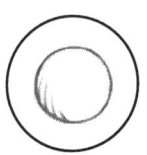

Form your flesh by exercising to *increase your physical capacity to act*.

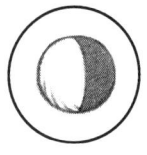

Divide the light from the darkness within by entering into the Lord's rest, eating whysely, and bridling your passions with exercise to *increase your physical capacity to practice self-mastery*.

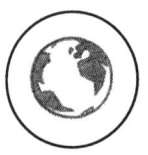

Beautify your fitness efforts by recreating your talents as you exercise to *increase your capacity to do good*.

Multiply the Blessings

LINE UPON LINE SUMMARY

Go!

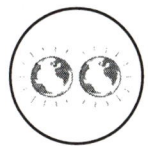 Multiply your fitness efforts by exercising to bless the life of another to *increase your physical capacity to experience a fulness of joy.*

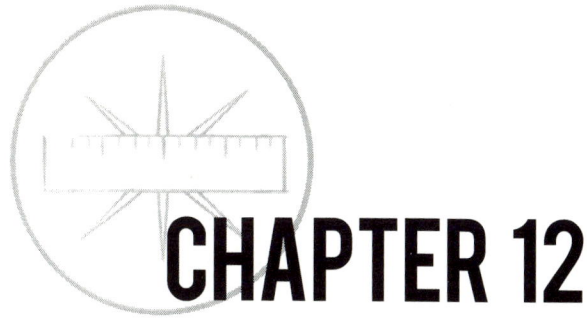

CHAPTER 12

Become Fit for Good

The momentum of the massive machine shook the ground beneath my feet. I could feel the vibrations move up my legs into my chest. "That's awesome," I exclaimed, as Tyler and I stood still, staring up at the biggest roller coaster we had ever seen. My family had moved next door to Tyler's family eight years previous. I knew my life would never be the same when I met him. He had Down's syndrome. Tyler and I became inseparable friends. We did everything together—from church to school to scouts. This particular summer, his parents had taken us to the only amusement park in Arizona for his sixteenth birthday.

"Let's ride that one first," I said, putting my arm around Tyler and pointing to the coaster.

He pulled my arm off his shoulder and shook his head. "No way! I'm not riding that thing. It's crazy!"

"Come on, Ty. We can tackle it, no problem," I replied.

The look on Tyler's face witnessed his commitment to keeping his feet on the ground.

I knew I had just dug myself into a hole with him, so I quickly changed the subject and challenged him to a round of bumper cars instead. He agreed. After giving each other a bad case of whiplash, we played several rounds of mini golf. We then ate lunch and worked our way up to the pirate boat that rocked back and forth, making our lunches creep ever so close to the surface. After the pirate ride, it was back to the bumper cars, always steering clear of the mammoth coaster. Our time was running out. In a couple of hours, Tyler's parents would take us home. I was determined to get Tyler to ride the coaster with me. So I turned to Tyler's hero for inspiration.

"Tyler, do you think Rocky could ride this coaster?" I asked.

"Come on, Rich," replied Tyler. "Of course he could!"

Tyler's childhood superhero was Rocky Balboa, a never-give-up and overcome-all-odds boxer featured in several movies in the 1980s. When we were younger, we loved to watch the Rocky movies. We loved them so much that as soon as we finished a movie we would wrap our knuckles with dishrags and go to the living room for a few rounds of boxing.

Like a ring announcer, I whispered in Tyler's ear, "In the far corner we have the world champion roller coaster, weighing in at two million tons . . . the amazing 'Desert Storm!'"

Tyler started to move his shoulders like a boxer warming up for a fight. I continued, "And in this corner, we have the challenger, weighing in at 149 pounds, a mass of muscle from Prescott, Arizona, . . . Rocky 'Tyler' Balboa!" Tyler raised his arms like a boxer and headed straight toward the coaster like a prizefighter to the ring.

"Yes!" I exclaimed, pumping my fist in excitement. "Let's do this, Rocky!"

We worked our way up through the maze of bars to the very front of the coaster. Tyler and I watched the coaster leave with a few riders and then return. He was quiet and focused. The gate opened. We entered the cart and pulled the safety bar over our laps. Tyler grabbed the bar and looked straight ahead. I could see the color in his hands fade to pale white as he gripped the safety bar tighter and tighter.

"Enjoy the ride," announced the attendant over the intercom. The coaster jerked forward and began its climb with a thunderous click . . . click . . . click.

Suddenly, Tyler turned to me with terror-filled eyes. "Rich, help!" he pleaded.

Become Fit for Good

"Tyler, are you all right?" I asked.

"No, I'm not!" he said, as tears began to form in his eyes. "I'm going to die!"

Tyler was serious. He had no doubt that this roller coaster was about to end his life. I waved my arms and yelled, trying in vain to get the attendant's attention. Our cart continued to climb up and up as Tyler became more and more terrified. His tears were now flowing down his face.

"Please stop the coaster!" he pleaded. I was powerless to help. I felt horrible for putting him in this situation. I tried my best to comfort him.

"Hold on tight," I said as I put my arms around him.

Click . . . click . . . click. The coaster continued to climb. We neared the peak of its upward climb. In a few seconds, we would drop over the edge to what Tyler thought was certain death. What happened next will be forever etched in my mind.

Tyler quickly let go of the safety bar, folded his arms, bowed his head, and prayed. He asked the Lord to spare his life. He quickly closed his sincere prayer in the name of his Savior just as the roller coaster began to crest over the edge. Time seemed to slow for me as the tears started to form in my eyes. I felt the Spirit settle in that coaster cart as it crept slowly over the edge, waiting for the carts behind to catch up and launch us into the massive loop.

At that moment, I saw Tyler become more than I ever imagined he could become. He quickly unfolded his arms, raised his hands high above his head, and screamed with absolute joy as we dropped into the loop. Not once did Tyler lower his hands as we bolted up, down, and around the track, eventually coming to a stop. I began to apologize for putting him in such a situation. He stopped me mid-sentence, and to my astonishment said, "Let's do it again!" We quickly exited the cart and raced back to the boarding area. For the next hour, we rode that roller coaster over and over again.

I still marvel at Tyler's transformation at the top of that coaster. In that moment, he was physically measured, yoked, and quickened by his relationship to his Father in Heaven, his faith in the Savior, and his connection to the Spirit. I was honored to see in that moment a glimpse of what he will *become* when the measure of his creation is filled with a fulness of eternal joy.

BECOME

I know of no other word that more perfectly captures the purpose of our creation than the word *become*. You are a spirit child of God. Like all offspring, you carry the genetic genes of your parents. You have the greatness of God within you, the divine DNA that defines your destiny to *become* like Him. This potential would have remained dormant in each of us had Adam and Eve not partaken of the forbidden fruit. The sacrifice of their immortality and presence with the Father provided our eternal spirits with a mortal body that would allow the fulness of our potential to be expressed. Remember, Adam fell that we might literally "be," meaning physical *be*-ings (see 2 Nephi 2:25). The coupling of our spirits with our mortal bodies is the "*be*" of our *be*coming like God.

In order for us to become like God, to fill the measure of our creation with joy, we must *come* unto Christ in order to be "changed from [our] carnal and fallen state, to a state of righteousness" and "become new creatures" in Christ (Mosiah 27:25–26). This change is called divine conversion, the "coming" process of be*coming* like God.

Divine conversion can be better understood when it is compared to the life-sustaining chemical conversions that take place within our bodies. A chemical reaction, like our conversion to become like God, requires three fundamental elements. The first is a *measured* physical substance that is capable of being acted upon and converted into something new. In the divine conversion process, the *measured* substance that God has given us to act upon is the elements of our bodies coupled with our spirit (see D&C 88:15). The second required element in a chemical reaction is the joining of the substance to an energy source that has sufficient power to complete the conversion process. In divine conversion, that power is found in the *yoke* of Christ, the priesthood ordinances that join us completely to the power of His Atonement, for His "grace is sufficient" to convert all of us (Ether 12:27). The third element in a chemical reaction is a catalyst. A catalyst is the element that helps *quicken* the conversion process. The catalyst of divine conversion in your life is the Holy Ghost, for when received He "shall . . . *quicken* your mortal bodies" to seal your divine conversion (Romans 8:11; emphasis added).

Conversion is a rebirth in which we are "born of the Spirit" (Moses 6:65) and "changed from [our] carnal and fallen state, to a state of righteousness" (Mosiah 27:25). That "state of righteousness" is a state of *becoming* "a new creature" in Christ (2 Corinthians 5:17) with the capacity to experience a fulness of joy, the purpose of our existence in this life and the next (see 2 Nephi 2:25). When resurrected in the next life, our spirits and bodies will be "inseparably connected," the connection that is required for us to "receive a fulness of joy" (D&C 93:33). Consider the words of Elder Bruce R. McConkie: "When the book of life is opened in the day of judgment (Revelation 20:12–15), men's *bodies* will show what law they have lived. The Great Judge will then read the record of the book of their lives; the account of their obedience or disobedience *will be written in their bodies*."[1]

Take a moment and ponder upon Elder McConkie's words. Our bodies are *becoming* the expressed image of our thoughts, words, and deeds (see Mosiah 4:30). Our bodies are the parchment that constitutes the book of life. All of God's children, "both old and young, both bond and free, both male and female, both the wicked and the righteous" will stand at the judgment bar with a perfected immortal body, free from all the diverse physical distortions, defects, and disabilities that can be experienced in mortality (Alma 11:43–44). However, the physical capacity of these perfected immortal bodies will vary. The Apostle Paul taught of this physical variation, "There are . . . celestial *bodies*, and *bodies* terrestrial: but the glory of the celestial is one, and the glory of the terrestrial is another. There is one glory of the sun, and another glory of the moon, and another glory of the stars: for one star differeth from another star in glory. So also is the resurrection of the dead" (1 Corinthians 15:40–42; emphasis added).

Fit for Good

What *is* the difference and what *makes* the difference between these resurrected bodies? We find the difference in their capacity to receive the glory of God. A celestial body *is* a body that is physically "prepared to stand the glory of the celestial kingdom"[2] and is a body that has the physical capacity to receive a "fulness of joy" (3 Nephi 28:10). What *makes* the difference between receiving a celestial, terrestrial, or telestial body? The answer is our degree of divine conversion we experience in this life—the degree to which we *become* a new creature in Christ, the degree that God's image has been "engraven upon [our] countenances" (Alma 5:19).

The adversary knows this. Every moment of his malicious existence is focused on disrupting your divine conversion in the "short time" he has during your mortal life (Revelation 12:12). He knows that he has absolutely no influence over the power source of divine conversion—the Atonement of Christ—or over the catalyst of divine conversion, his opposite in spirit, the Holy Ghost.

Therefore, the way Satan can confound your divine conversion is to focus his efforts upon the substance of that conversion, the mortal elements that he so desperately desires but will never have—the elements that constitute your physical body. He knows that if he can limit your *physical capacity to act, to practice self-mastery, to do good*, and *to experience a fulness of joy*, he can hinder or halt your divine conversion. He knows that the degree to which he can limit your divine conversion in this life is the degree to which he can limit your eternal potential in the life to come (see Alma 41:12–15).

This is why it is important that we understand the eternal principles, practices, and patterns that will enable us to exercise righteous dominion over the elements of our bodies.

Consider the young mother who decides to get physically *fit for good*. She internalizes the doctrine that helps her step to the eternal marks and get set for the opposition of exercise. She creates her fitness focus statement and asks her husband to be her fitness fellow. Together, they measure her initial capacity to act and score and then record it on her Fitness Focus Sphere that they put on the fridge. She commits to allow more light into

Become Fit for Good

her life by doing her best to enter the rest of the Lord for at least six hours each night, to be whyse in what she eats, and to exercise at least five days a week to help her bridle her natural passions.

After learning that her current exercise preference is social, spontaneous, and collaborative, she decides to enlarge her talent for dance by attending the extremely early-morning exercise dance class put on by the stake Relief Society. She magnifies her fitness focus by focusing her efforts on exercising to bless her boys with a mother who is slow to anger.

For the first few weeks, her body protests the 5:00 a.m. wake-up call. However, she finds strength each time she kneels in prayer to invite the Spirit to be with her and to consecrate her efforts before she heads out to the stake center.

She enjoys being with her friends each morning as they exercise together in their various degrees of morning glory. As she exercises, her brain sends impulses of light throughout her body, which cause her heart rate and blood pressure to rise, her pupils to dilate, and her neck hair to rise. She knows that each bout of exercise serves as a mini wilderness experience in which the fallen elements of her body are waxing strong under the dominion of her divine spirit. At the end of the dance class, she feels energized, ready to go home and care for her little ones.

She returns home and whysely chooses to make whole-wheat pancakes for her family. She steps away from the pancakes for a moment, only to return to find that her twin boys are flinging the flour at each other. Her heart rate and blood pressure rise. Her pupils dilate as the hair on the back of her neck rises. The fallen elements of her body are perfectly primed to lash out in anger at her boys. However, she recognizes this feeling and remembers her fitness focus and the dominion she gained over the elements of her body earlier that morning. With a deep breath, she bridles her anger and calmly separates her two boys. She then informs them with a kind but firm voice that breakfast will be delayed until they clean the kitchen. Stunned by her masterful reaction, the twins quickly obey. Their mother smiles as she feels the exponential joy of blessing her boys by *becoming*, at least in that moment, a new creature in Christ, a mother who was slow to anger.

WIN!

I love the words attributed to Sadie Tiller Crawley:

> He stood at the crossroads all alone,
> The sunlight on his face.
> He had no thought for the world unknown—
> He was set for a manly race.
> But the roads stretched east and the roads stretched west,
> And the lad knew not which road was best.
> So he chose the road that led him down,
> And he lost the race and the victor's crown.
> He was caught at last in an angry snare
> Because no one stood at the crossroads there
> To show him the better road
>
> Another day at the self-same place
> A boy with high hopes stood.
> He, too, was set for a manly race;
> He, too, was seeking the things that were good.
> But one was there whom the roads did know,
> And that one showed him which way to go.
> So he turned from the road that would lead him down,
> And he won the race and the victor's crown.
> He walks today the highway fair
> Because one stood at the crossroads there
> To show him the better way.[3]

You now know that there is a better, "more excellent way" (1 Corinthians 12:31) to improve your physical fitness that is founded upon true doctrine. True doctrine that, when "understood," will improve your fitness behavior "quicker than the study of behavior will."[4] Over the last twelve chapters, you have been introduced to the doctrinal principles, patterns, and practices that can increase your physical capacity to run the race of life (see 1 Corinthians 9:24) so that you might "win the prize" (Mosiah 4:27)—the eternal gift (see D&C 14:7) that will enable you to you *become* physically *fit for good,* and to have the physical capacity to do good forever, like God.

Become Fit for Good

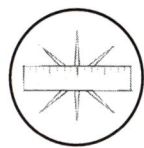 You are a child of God. Through the measure of your creation, the yoke of Christ, and the quickening of the Spirit, you can *become* physically *fit for good*—like Him.

LINE UPON LINE SUMMARY

On Your Mark

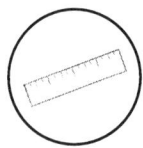

Receive God's image. Remember, your body is *the measure of your creation*—the physical manifestation of your potential to become like God.

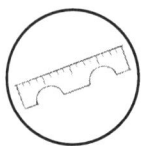

Yoke yourself to Christ when you exercise. Remember, *His yoke will enable* the measure of your creation to be filled with a fulness of joy.

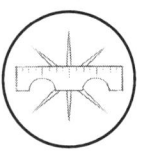

Invite the Spirit to be with you when you exercise. Remember, *His power will quicken* the measure of your creation so you can experience a fulness of joy.

LINE UPON LINE SUMMARY

Get Set

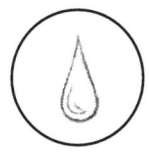
Sweat in the wilderness of regular exercise. The *sweat of your brow* is the manifestation of your effort to subject the fallen elements of your body to your divine spirit.

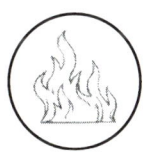
Defend against the adversary's fiery darts. *Watch and pray* for protection against the darts of physical lust, latency, and limits that will fill the measure of your creation with misery.

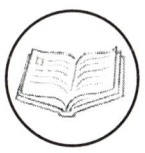
Experiment upon the word of God. By *exercising faith in the word of God*, you can increase your physical capacity to fill the measure of your creation with a fulness of joy.

Fit for Good

LINE UPON LINE SUMMARY

Go!

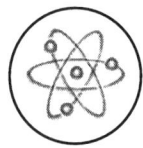

Create a *fitness focus statement*. Select a *fitness fellow* to return and report to about your efforts to claim the blessings of exercising according to the Lord's pattern of creation.

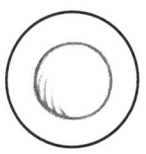

Form your flesh by exercising to *increase your physical capacity to act*.

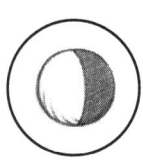

Divide the light from the darkness within by entering into the Lord's rest, eating whysely, and bridling your passions with exercise to *increase your physical capacity to practice self-mastery*.

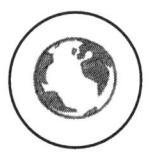

Beautify your fitness efforts by recreating your talents as you exercise to *increase your capacity to do good*.

LINE UPON LINE SUMMARY

Go!

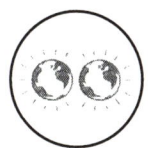

Multiply your fitness efforts by exercising to bless the life of another to *increase your physical capacity to experience a fulness of joy.*

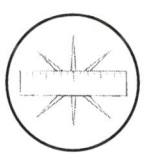

You are a child of God. Through the measure of your creation, the yoke of Christ, and the quickening of the Spirit, you can *become* physically *fit for good*—like Him.

NOTES

Preface

1. Henry B Eyring, "Help Them on Their Way Home," *Ensign*, May 2010.
2. Dieter F. Uchtdorf, "Waiting on the Road to Damascus," *Ensign*, May 2011.
3. Boyd K. Packer, "Little Children," *Ensign*, November 1986.
4. Dieter F. Uchtdorf, "Waiting on the Road to Damascus," *Ensign*, May 2011.

Introduction

1. Elizabeth Mendes, "Americans Exercising Slightly More in 2012," *Gallup*, September 19, 2012; www.gallup.com/poll/157505/americans-exercising-slightly-2012.aspx.
2. Boyd K. Packer, "Little Children," *Ensign*, November 1986.

Chapter 1

1. *Brigham Young, Discourses of Brigham Young*, selected by John A. Widtsoe (Salt Lake City: Deseret Book, 1925), 78; emphasis added.

Notes

2. Elaine S. Dalton, "Remember Who You Are!," *Ensign*, May 2010; emphasis added.
3. Dieter F. Uchtdorf, "Of Things That Matter Most," *Ensign*, November 2010.
4. Russell M. Nelson, "'Joy Cometh in the Morning,'" *Ensign*, November 1986; emphasis added.
5. *Brigham Young, Discourses of Brigham Young*, selected by John A. Widtsoe (Salt Lake City: Deseret Book, 1925), 78.

Chapter 2

1. David A. Bednar, "Bear Up Their Burdens with Ease," *Ensign*, May 2014.
2. David O. McKay, *Pathways to Happiness*, comp. Llewelyn R. McKay (Salt Lake City: Bookcraft, 1957).

Chapter 3

1. Bruce R. McConkie, *Mormon Doctrine*, 2nd ed., s.v. "transfiguration" (Salt Lake City: Bookcraft, 1979), 803.
2. Guide to the Scriptures, "Quicken"; scriptures.lds.org
3. Parley P. Pratt, *Key to the Science of Theology*, 7th ed. (Deseret Book, 1915), 95–96.
4. Richard G. Scott, "How to Obtain Revelation and Inspiration for Your Personal Life," *Ensign*, May 2012.
5. "Frequently Asked Questions: Why is it important for us to take care of our bodies? Why are our bodies called temples of God in the Bible?," *Mormon.org*, https://www.mormon.org.au/faq/topic/health/question/care-for-our-bodies.
6. Parley P. Pratt, *Key to the Science of Theology*, 7th ed. (Deseret Book, 1915), 95–96; emphasis added.

Notes

Chapter 4

1. James E. Talmage, *Jesus the Christ* (Salt Lake City: Deseret Book, 1915), 199.

Chapter 5

1. David A. Bednar, "Things as They Really Are," *Ensign*, June 2010.
2. Ibid.
3. Ibid.
4. Ryan Jaslow, "CDC: 80 percent of American adults don't get recommended exercise," *CBS News*, May 3, 2013.

Chapter 6

1. *Lectures on Faith* (Salt Lake City: Deseret Book, 1985), 11–12; emphasis added.
2. Stuart Wolpert, "Dieting Does Not Work, UCLA Researchers Report," *UCLA Newsroom*, April 3, 2007, http://newsroom.ucla.edu/releases/Dieting-Does-Not-Work-UCLA-Researchers-7832.
3. *Lectures on Faith* (Salt Lake City: Deseret Book, 1985), 58–59; emphasis added.
4. James E. Talmage, *Jesus the Christ* (Salt Lake City: Deseret Book, 1915), 199.

Chapter 7

1. David O. McKay, *Pathways to Happiness*, comp. Llewelyn R. McKay (Salt Lake City: Bookcraft, 1957), xi; emphasis added.
2. Dieter F. Uchtdorf, "Happiness, Your Heritage," *Ensign*, November 2008; emphasis added.
3. Jeffrey R. Holland, "The Call to Be Christlike," *Ensign*, June 2014.
4. Dieter F. Uchtdorf, "Tending the Flock: Teaching Leadership Skills to Youth," *Ensign*, June 2008; emphasis added.

Notes

5. Thomas S. Monson, in Conference Report, October 1970, 107; emphasis added.
6. Neal A. Maxwell, "Jesus, the Perfect Mentor," *Ensign*, February 2001.
7. Russell M. Nelson, "Decisions for Eternity," *Ensign*, October 2013.

Chapter 9

1. *Lectures on Faith* (Salt Lake City: Deseret Book, 1985); emphasis added.
2. "Why Do We Sleep, Anyway?," *Harvard Medical School*, last reviewed December 18, 2007; http://healthysleep.med.harvard.edu/healthy/matters/benefits-of-sleep/why-do-we-sleep.
3. "How Much Sleep Do We Really Need?," *National Sleep Foundation*, http://sleepfoundation.org/how-sleep-works/how-much-sleep-do-we-really-need.
4. Ibid.

Chapter 10

1. Richard G. Scott, "Finding Joy in Life," *Ensign*, May 1996.
2. D. Todd Christofferson, "Reflections on a Consecrated Life," *Ensign*, November 2010; emphasis added.
3. Dieter F. Uchtdorf, "Happiness, Your Heritage," *Ensign*, November 2008.

Chapter 11

1. "NTSB/AAR-82/08: Aircraft Accident Report—Air Florida, Inc., Boeing 737-222, N62AF, Collision with 14th Street Bridge, Near Washington National Airport, Washington, D.C., January 13, 1982," *National Transportation Safety Board*, January 13, 1982, 21–22; http://libraryonline.erau.edu/online-full-text/ntsb/aircraft-accident-reports/AAR82-08.pdf.

Notes

2. Roger Rosenblatt, "The Man in the Water," *Time Magazine*, January 25, 1982.

Chapter 12

1. Bruce R. McConkie, *Mormon Doctrine*, 2nd ed., s.v. "transfiguration" (Salt Lake City: Bookcraft, 1979), 97; emphasis added.
2. Bruce R. McConkie, "The Dead Who Die in the Lord," *Ensign*, November 1976.
3. Sadie Tiller Crawley, "At the Crossroads," in *Best-Loved Poems of the LDS People*, ed. Jack M. Lyon and Linda Ririe Gundry (Salt Lake City: Deseret Book, 1996), 313. See also Thomas S. Monson, "Your Jericho Road," *Ensign*, February 1989.
4. Boyd K. Packer, "Little Children," *Ensign*, November 1986.

PERSONAL NOTES

Record your thoughts and experiences as you become fit for good.

Personal Notes

Personal Notes

Personal Notes

Personal Notes

Personal Notes

Personal Notes

Personal Notes

Personal Notes

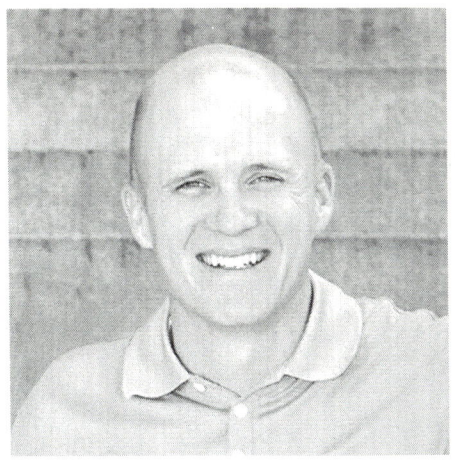

ABOUT THE AUTHOR
Dr. H. Rich Tenney

Dr. H. Rich Tenney received his doctor of physical therapy degree with honors from Elon University in 2006. Dr. Tenney is a certified postural restoration specialist, as well as a health and wellness coach. His physical therapy research has been presented and published on national and international levels. He is a former seminary teacher and bishop, and is currently serving as a member of the stake presidency in Prescott, Arizona, where he lives with his wife and four children.

Scan to visit

www.physicallyfitforgood.com

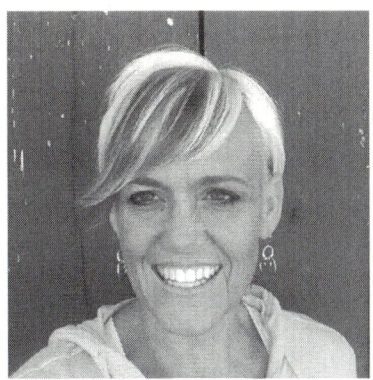

ABOUT THE AUTHOR

Liz Tennyson

Liz Tennyson is an author, speaker, and success mentor in the areas of life, health, and online business strategy. As a multi-passionate entrepreneur, she uses her gift as a multiplier to help others quickly transform and stretch their capacity for growth. She loves running women's retreats for a total immersion experience that helps facilitate life change. She runs the organization The Fit Mormon Life.

Her top priority is her family. Married to her husband Toby for nineteen years, they have four children that each provide unique blessings to the family.

Liz loves God and the Savior. She lives a radical life of service and loves making friends everywhere she goes.

Scan to visit

www.imafitmormon.org